PERVASIVE HEALTHCARE COMPUTING

T0142988

PERVASIVE HEALTHCARE COMPUTING:
EMR/EHR, WIRELESS and HEALTH MONITORING

Upkar Varshney

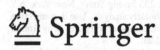 Springer

Upkar Varshney
Georgia State University
Atlanta, GA
USA

ISBN: 978-1-4419-5496-1   e-ISBN: 978-1-4419-0215-3
DOI: 10.1007/978-1-4419-0215-3

© Springer Science+Business Media, LLC 2010
All rights reserved. This work may not be translated or copied in whole or in part without the written permission of the publisher (Springer Science+Business Media, LLC, 233 Spring Street, New York, NY 10013, USA), except for brief excerpts in connection with reviews or scholarly analysis. Use in connection with any form of information storage and retrieval, electronic adaptation, computer software, or by similar or dissimilar methodology now known or hereafter developed is forbidden.
The use in this publication of trade names, trademarks, service marks, and similar terms, even if they are not identified as such, is not to be taken as an expression of opinion as to whether or not they are subject to proprietary rights.

Printed on acid-free paper

9 8 7 6 5 4 3 2 1

springer.com

The book is dedicated to
My parents
Vimala Kumari and L. P. Varshney
&
My wife
Smita Varshney

Acknowledgments

As a professor, I am very thankful to my doctoral and graduate students. I would also like to acknowledge the support I have received from National Science Foundation.

I would like to especially thank students of my Pervasive Healthcare Technologies course during Fall 2008 at GSU for their support. These students include Philip Burns, Tabitha Carney, John Crane, Clifford Eiche, Dwight Elliston, Vinu Jose, Andrew Katz, David Laird, Ebakole Osara, David Redmond, Kavipriya Shanmugam, Yung-yu Su, Sanchitha Suresh, and Mary Walters.

I should most sincerely thank my wife Smita. This book would not be possible without her inspiration and constant support. I also owe a lot to my two daughters Juhi and Jaaie, who have been very supportive throughout the book writing process.

Finally, I should also thank the people at Springer, including Amy Brais, Jennifer Evans and Kelly Moritz for their help in getting the book published.

Upkar Varshney
Georgia State University

Pervasive Healthcare Computing

List of Contents

CHAPTER 1 Healthcare Systems: Challenges and Solutions

Abstract In this chapter, we address the functioning and limitations of existing healthcare system systems. More specifically, we address healthcare in the US and examine its strengths and challenges. To improve the current healthcare systems, first several general solutions are presented. Then, several technology-oriented solutions are introduced and discussed. Finally, how the rest of the book is organized in terms of covered topics, is presented.

1.1 Healthcare System in US

The healthcare system is unique due to its focus on human care and the regulatory environment it has to operate in. The current situation is fairly complex in the US. On one hand, the US spends the most amount of money per person on healthcare in the world [1], it also has a large number of uninsured people totaling about 47 million or 16% of the population [2]. It would need about $100 Billion/year to the healthcare expenses if everyone is insured. Several international studies rank US healthcare system very high in responsiveness and emergency care, but lower in efficiencies and performance, level of infant mortality, overall health quality, life expectancy and number of preventable deaths.

There is a lack of focus on preventive care, widespread obesity and patients with multiple chronic problems, shortage of healthcare professionals, inefficiencies in healthcare delivery, overpriced medications and poor adherence, large number of medical mistakes and quality of care challenges, and lack of technologies and access to information. The US healthcare system is always touted as "patient-centric", but a myriad of rules, regulations and problems lead to a situation where some patients receive more than necessary care while others receive little to no care. Some of these differences are based on economic disparity, location, and the current employment. There are controls on who can receive service and who can not. A large number of players such as healthcare professionals, hospitals, insurance companies, drug manufactures, and lawyers also make patient care even more complex.

The situation is quite different from other western countries where governments are much more involved in universal healthcare, directly employing physicians and healthcare professionals, putting price control on medications and healthcare services, limiting malpractice lawsuits, and focusing on expensive preventive care.

U. Varshney, *Pervasive Healthcare Computing: EMR/EHR, Wireless and Health Monitoring*,
DOI: 10.1007/978-1-4419-0215-3_1,
© Springer Science + Business Media, LLC 2009

In many of these countries, health technology adoption is also very significant due to the government mandates funded by higher taxes.

Next, we present several challenges faced by the US healthcare system and discuss possible solutions one by one.

1.2 Costs and Complexity of Payments

In the US, the total healthcare spending from all public and private sources reached $2.1 trillion dollars in 2006, with major components shown on Table 1 [3]. The government is the largest payer, accounting for slightly less than half of the direct expenses. Assuming no major changes in the current healthcare policies, the cost of healthcare services is expected to rise to 20% of the US GDP by 2015 with an estimated annual growth of about 7%. The government is expected to pay about half of the healthcare bill in 2015, and if tax subsidies are also included, the number would go up by another $200 Billion/year.

Several factors have contributed to this rise including longer life spans, breakthroughs in medical technology and rising incomes, unhealthy life styles, lack of health promotional programs, limited adherence to medications, and high-stress in work places and daily life. Also, an increasing number of people, such as baby boomers, have become eligible for coverage through Medicare (the federal health program for the elderly) and Medicaid for people with low incomes. With rising incomes, some people are willing to spend more money for staying healthy. This may translate into more research and development of new, costly medical technologies and medications, which increases the healthcare cost. The current medicine is also based on extending the human life as much as possible, even when the quality of life for the patient is decreasing significantly.

Table 1.1 Healthcare costs and major components

Item	Amount in $Billions	Percent of total health-care cost	Estimated future growth (2008-2017)
Hospital care	648	30.86	7%
Physician and clinical services	660	31.43	6.5%
Home Health	53	2.52	7.5%
Nursing Home Health	125	5.95	5.2%
Prescription drugs	217	10.33	8%
Other medical products	59	2.81	4%
Program administration	145	6.90	7%
Government Public Health Activities	59	2.81	7%
Investment (research and infrastructure)	139	6.62	6%

There are several health insurance plans and payers in the US healthcare system. These include government's Medicaid for poor and handicapped people, private insurance plans primarily for working and self-employed people younger than 65, and government's Medicare for people 65 and older. In addition, there are many special insurance plans for federal government employees and veterans. Out of all healthcare expenses, private insurance plans cover about 34%, Medicare 19%, Medicaid 15%, other public plans 12%, patients 12%, and other private sources covered 7% [10]. The premiums for private insurance plans are paid by employers and employees in some combinations. There are a few controls on how much a private insurance plan may cost, although some employers may be able to negotiate some rates in exchange for some restrictions and healthcare coverage levels. Some states, such as Massachusetts, have been able to create state-wide universal coverage, but the nationwide universal coverage does not exist in the US. There has been a lot of discussion on how to move towards universal coverage. Some of the health plans under discussion range from single-payer plan to continuation of existing healthcare plans with tax-subsidies for insurance premiums of currently uninsured people.

In the multi-player healthcare system, everyone should be asked to more aggressively manage the rising cost and this will reduce the growth of overall cost by a large percentage. There are several ways to cut costs including significant reduction in bureaucracy, reducing the growth of salaries of physicians and CEOs and/or matching it to the quality of care, and by reducing the cost of medical supplies and drugs. Any such savings should be encouraged to be invested in suitable healthcare infrastructure, which enhances the efficiency of healthcare delivery and could reduce the future cost of healthcare. The investment in suitable infrastructure will also increase the effectiveness of medical care. The government should increase investment in various processes and methods which can make the delivery of healthcare more efficient while reducing the number of medical errors.

1.3 Limited Number of Healthcare Professionals

The current regulatory environment limits how many physicians can be trained and employed in the US. The number of physicians graduating from the US medical schools has not increased much since 1980s. For example, 15632 doctors graduated in 1980-81 and 15712 in 2000-01 [6]. During this time, the US population has increased 24% from 226 million to 281 million. For many reasons, the level of complexity is so enormous that it is almost impossible for a new medical school to start or an existing one to train more medical students. Also, many physicians choose to practice in urban or suburban areas due to income, family, and other reasons. This ensures that there is always a shortage of physicians in many places, resulting in very high salary for physicians. Many physicians carry large loans taken for completing their expensive medical training, and thus are much more influenced by financial considerations. The compensation for physicians alone represents about 20% of all healthcare expenses in the US and could range from $100K-$500K, with median closer to $200K [8]. Additionally, more physicians choose specialties with higher income potential, thus limiting the number of physicians in lower-paying primary care areas. This will have major impact on the general health of the nation as receiving preventive care would become even more difficult in the future.

The situation is quite different for other healthcare professionals, such as nurses, pharmacists, technicians, physician assistants and physical therapists. There is also some shortage of these professionals and as many of the allied health schools in the US primarily offer advanced and terminal degrees in such fields, the salaries of these healthcare professionals have also been increasing. For nurses, many obstacles have been reduced in the training, licensing, and employment for both US born and internationally trained. The annual compensation of nurses ranges from $40K to $100K, higher for head of nursing.

While the supply of some healthcare professionals is limited, the quality of training is generally very good with strict certifications and licensing requirements. Some individual decisions about entering healthcare profession are influenced by monetary concerns more than the quality of patient care. Some healthcare professionals are also influenced by the amount of money drug companies have put in the advertisement, training and speaker's honorariums. The cost of doing business has also been rising for physicians, thus affecting their attitude towards patients care. The increasing potential for malpractice law-suits has also increased the cost of malpractice insurance, resulting in further increased cost of doing business. To manage these, several reforms, including peer-review of medical errors, as opposed to judicial trial, for determining patient harm and reimbursements, have been proposed and are under consideration in different states in the US. The quality of life for healthcare professionals has been dropping and more specifically, being a physician is no longer the same career charm for younger people and their parents in the US.

In general, increasing the number of healthcare professionals will improve the quality of care with reduced patient load, will improve access to healthcare professionals for preventive care, and will reduce the number of medical errors. The supply and demand of healthcare professionals should be addressed on a long-term basis by healthcare entities and various governments. There are several ways to address this by increasing the number of medical and allied health schools, number of students enrolled per school and the number of foreign healthcare professionals who can be trained in the US hospitals. These can also be facilitated by simplifying the various regulatory processes and removing current procedural hurdles. The need to add more faculty at medical and allied health schools should also be addressed along with necessary medical and educational technologies to maintain the quality of training for healthcare professionals. Also, the US government needs to be more proactive in increasing the funding for medical training and encouraging more foreign doctors who are completing medical residencies in the US to stay here by simplifying the visa and waiver processes. For many medical specialties with shortage of physicians, US government could add more scholarships and other financial incentives including low interest loans to increase the supply.

1.4 Technological & Other Inefficiencies in Healthcare

There are several technological and other inefficiencies in healthcare services. These include the use of paper-based system for patient records, the use of little to no technology to out-dated technology, and, delivery of unnecessary care to avoid malpractice law-suits. The factors that sometimes affect the introduction and adoption of technologies generally include lack of funding, possible disruption of care, and dealing with learning curve before technologies are usable in fast-paced medical care. The "defensive medicine" leads to many expensive services, procedures and treatments that may not be necessary. There are also inefficiencies in how the care is provided such as an expert seeing a patient with minor health problems. There is also a lack of preventive care, use of emergency rooms to get access to necessary non-emergency care, and discontinuation of care after symptoms fade away.

In general, hospitals in the US have many challenges. They can not deny services to patients, even those with no insurance, in cases of emergencies, but could transfer them to another location once the patient is stabilized. In case of regular care, a hospital may deny care or require part of the payments if insurance plan does not exist or cover the needed healthcare services. The capacity of most hospitals is based on government or state regulations, which include the needs-assessment in the process of giving permission to new hospitals or allowing existing hospitals to expand. A vast majority of rooms in hospitals are underused in normal conditions. This does increase the per-room cost when patients stay in the hospitals. The cost of stay in a US hospital ranges from $3000 to $10,000/day. Although, it is claimed that hospital rooms would be needed in case of disasters and unusual circumstances, these are not enough even for a small disaster affecting a few thousand people. Also, many nursing homes are operated with inefficiencies in terms of older technologies and use of excess staff for periodic observation of the patients. The cost of keeping a patient in a nursing home in the US is about $40K per year, majority of which is paid by Medicare and the rest by patients and their families.

In addition to all the above, bureaucracy in healthcare is eating up 35% of all healthcare dollars. This includes the administrative cost for hospitals, doctors' office, and insurance companies. This is one major area where IT and wireless technologies can significantly cut the cost of healthcare. More specifically, universal accessibility to electronic medical records will reduce the long-term cost of healthcare services. Implementation of simpler and more efficient processes such as those in automated and simplified billing for services could also reduce the administrative cost. Simplifying the health laws could reduce the number of malpractice suits and thus the extent of defensive medicine and malpractice premiums for healthcare professionals.

1.5 Patients-related Challenges

Chronic diseases, which do not have a cure but could lead to major adverse events and complications for patients, are a major part of US healthcare system. The most common chronic diseases are cancers, hypertension, diabetes, stroke, mental disorders, heart diseases, and asthma affecting about half of the US population. To make things even worse, some of the patients, known as high risk patients, have multiple chronic diseases. According to an estimate, about 8 million of Medicare patients with five or more chronic conditions account for 76% of all healthcare expenses [12]. Also, 92% of the Medicare expenses were by patients with three or more chronic diseases [12].

Within US, most people view health conditions, including weight problems, as a private issue and with busier life styles and high stress, they are not able to address these challenges. A lack of exercise, more sedentary life styles, richer and processed diets, and higher stress are all affecting the number of people with weight problems. The level of obesity has been rising since 1980s and has reached to 34% among all adults, however the level is shown to be stabilizing since 2004 [13]. When these adults move to their geriatric years, their healthcare needs will be significantly higher than today's elderly. This would lead to continuous growth in patients with one or more chronic illnesses. The number of such patients is only estimated to grow higher with an exponential increase in the number of seniors and retirees in the current baby boomer's generation (the people born between 1946 and 1964 in the US). This would lead to significant increase in the healthcare cost. There are also some more patients-related challenges in the healthcare needs of a large number of people who have served/serving in the armed forces. Although estimates vary, about 100,000 people will require long-term care for physical and mental injuries received in the recent wars.

In addition, many patients in the US have high expectations from healthcare providers in receiving immediate, world class, and comprehensive customer service, even for minor problems. This combines with the ability to sue anyone anytime anywhere in case anything unexpected and/or unusual happens, increase the complexity of healthcare challenges even more.

One of the solutions of the above problems is Proactive health, which can be defined as the level of health and wellness received, when patients, families, healthcare professionals, governments and insurance companies work together. To achieve proactive health, several steps are necessary. This includes creating a much higher level of health-awareness in the society covering children, adults, and older consumers. Creating an awareness of unhealthy life styles and restricting access to unhealthy food items is an important step. There should also be financial incentives for health wellness and health maintenance. The city, state and federal governments must invest in public infrastructure to encourage walking, biking and more physical activities. The cost of regular checkups and preventive care should be very minimal. The basic theme here is to invest in the overall health today to cut down the cost tomorrow. The proactive health should reduce the incidence of one or multiple chronic conditions. And, even when such conditions occur, the chronic conditions can be managed better by a combination of patient compliance and life style changes.

1.6 Cost of Medications & Poor Adherence

One of the major components of healthcare expenses is the cost of prescription medications. To start with, this is related to the cost of research and development, which is claimed to be close to $1Billion for a successful drug that is Food and Drug Administration (FDA) approved. Although, some researchers estimate the total cost of developing a drug to be in the range of $200-500m. The manufacturing, distribution and marketing processes, including the use of hiring practicing physicians as expert speakers, add another layer of cost. Since currently there is no cost-control on what drug companies can charge for medications in the US, the cost has been rising at a faster rate than the rate of inflation. The use of generic medications does reduce the cost, however, these are normally available to public only after the patent on the drug expires. Some pharmaceuticals are trying to file for additional patents for competitive advantages and thus could delay the availability of generic drugs. In many western countries not including the US, the governments negotiate the price of various medications or use a range of price controls on what could be charged by pharmaceuticals.

In addition to the cost of medications, the other major problem is partial compliance to medications, where patients do not follow the prescribed regimen. It has been estimated that only about one third of all patients take their prescription medications regularly. There may be several reasons behind such limited adherence including patients' fear of potential side-effects, the need to cut their out-of-pocket cost for medications, and the assumption that they are fine and thus no longer need to continue. This lack of adherence results in increased morbidity and disease related complications, thus requiring further hospitalization and added cost of healthcare. Some information technologies can help in increasing the level of adherence to medications by using reminders (alarms), and by monitoring the use of medications including those of addictive nature. The health insurance companies could provide incentives to these patients for improved adherence for better health, which may reduce the future healthcare expenses to be paid by the insurance companies.

1.7 Medical Errors & Quality of Care

Every year, many medical errors occur in the US resulting in hundreds of thousands of deaths and injuries. According to a report from the Institute of Medicine, somewhere between 44,000 to 98,000 people die in US hospitals every year due to medical errors [14]. The report recommended that voluntary and mandatory error reporting programs should be created, measures should be taken to improve patient safety, and failures of various systems should be addressed. It may be years, if not decade, before such interventions are put in place to better manage the number of medical errors.

The most common medical errors in general practice are investigation errors, errors in diagnosis, treatment errors, communication errors, and errors in office administration [11]. The frequency and impact of medical errors are likely to be different in specialized practices and hospitals. Although the quality of care in general is very good at US hospitals, but according to a CDC report, about 7% of emergency room visits involve patients who have been recently discharged from hospitals [9]. This raises questions on both the prior care and the follow-up care after the hospital discharge.

Some medical errors, possibly resulting in wrong diagnosis and drug interaction problems, occur due to a lack of correct and complete information at the location and time it is needed. The current load and considerable stress on healthcare professionals also contributes to medical mistakes. The use of IT and wireless technologies can significantly reduce the number of medical errors, possibly saving many lives and considerable healthcare cost. There should be incentives to hospitals, doctors, and insurance companies, and patients for delivering or receiving the best possible quality of care and also for performance and efficiencies.

There is some momentum on payments for better care, which may reduce the future occurrence of episodes and thus healthcare expenses for the patients. Currently, payments are made for healthcare services including those involving medical mistakes. Ideally, there should be no payments for such medical mistakes and there is some momentum in Medicare and private insurance companies towards no payment if a medical mistake is made in the covered procedure or treatment. In such cases, patients should also not be expected to pay anything. Many states are proposing rules to stop hospitals and physicians from submitting claims for treatment affected by medical errors.

The follow up care could be improved to reduce the recovery time and also to reduce future hospitalizations. More work can also be done towards continuous improvement in healthcare delivery by focusing on the delivery process, reduction in medical mistakes, and improvement in the quality of care.

1.8 Healthcare Billing and Fraud

The current healthcare billing system is complex and prone to errors. Typically, hospitals and physicians submit one or more codes for the service delivered. These requests are checked for the medically necessary care and reasonable cost. The sheer number of codes and varying interpretation of which codes to use for what services lead to many errors and in some cases even on-purpose fraudulent charges in the billing for healthcare services.

To start with, the billing for healthcare services could be simplified, thus allowing more automated processes to check for necessary service and suitable charges, to reduce the administrative cost. More efforts are also needed in fraud detection and prevention. In general, a vast majority of healthcare services involve correct and honest charges, but some level of fraud does exist in the healthcare system. It is believed that majority of bills contain errors including fraudulent charges. This only increases the amount of time and efforts that must be spent in verifying and analyzing medical bills by public and private insurance companies. This adds to the administrative cost of healthcare in the US.

More work is needed in automated detection of fraud in healthcare services and billing and there should be more stiff penalties for any healthcare fraud. New automated algorithms and computer programs can be deployed to verify the codes for payments along with claims of time spent in the care. If someone is claiming to see 20 patients for 40 minutes each in an 8-hour day, the automated fraud detection system can easily detect the exaggerated claims for service by adding the total time from all the codes to check. More sophisticated systems could be designed and employed to detect presence of unnecessary procedures and treatments by processing patient's history and current conditions.

1.9 Improvements with Technologies in Healthcare

As discussed, several changes could be made to the current healthcare system to increase its effectiveness while reducing the healthcare cost. More work is needed in comparing the relative effectiveness of the proposed solutions in sections 1.2-1.8. Some of the changes can be introduced in one step, while others may be introduced more gradually.

In this book, we focus on how technologies, especially information and communications technologies, can help improve healthcare systems worldwide. In general, these technologies can allow information to be available anywhere any time to anyone authorized, make the delivery of healthcare services more efficient, by reducing the number of tasks that need to be done by healthcare professionals, and encourage and motivate patients to take better control of their healthcare needs and life style. One of the objectives is to show how technologies can lead to the desired evolution of healthcare system as shown in Figure 1.1. It should be noted that technologies alone can not create all the necessary changes, but the involvement of various stakeholders and patients is necessary for such evolution of healthcare system. There are certain cultural and organizational characteristics of healthcare systems that may assist in such evolution. These include the "can do" attitude and individualism of people, which could add to the adoption of various technologies for more independent living.

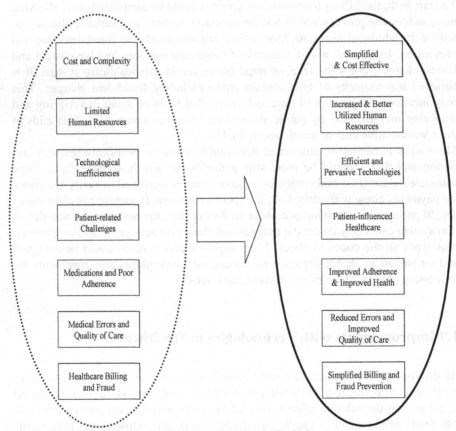

Fig. 1.1 The Present Healthcare System and Desirable Evolution

1.9.1 Use of Technological Advances

There are several suitable information and communications technologies for healthcare. These could be divided among four categories: implanted (inside human body), wearable, portable, and environmental. The use of implanted technologies could include use of Radio Frequency Identification (RFID) and sensors inside the human body. Normally, RFID chips would store medical and other information, while sensors could measure one or more medical parameters. The wearable technologies include the use of Smart Shirts, which are designed to wear for extended period of time for monitoring of health conditions. These shirts with attached sensors could be washed, ironed and charged for use. In future, these could be networked with other devices and people. The portable devices, such as handheld computers and phones, can be used in monitoring and recording health conditions. Finally, environmental technologies include adding computing and communications capabilities in the surrounding of patients. An example is "Smart" Home, where appliances have smartness to assist people in their daily activities. Additionally, telemedicine and mobile telemedicine technologies can be used to improve the overall quality of care. The decision to use one or more categories of technologies would be best served by including patient's conditions, preferences, comfort, safety and cost.

1.9.2 Anytime Anywhere Access to Medical Information

Some medical errors, possibly resulting in wrong diagnosis and drug interaction problems, occur due to a lack of correct and complete information at the location and time it is needed. Using a richer environment of information and communications technologies, the medical information can be made available at "any place anytime" using sophisticated devices and widely deployed networks. Electronic Medical Records (EMRs) or Electronic Health Records (EHRs) with detailed patient information can be accessed anywhere anytime by anyone who is authorized. Although not all medical errors can be eliminated, but some informational-errors can be avoided by "anytime anywhere" access to medical information. The overall quality and healthcare coverage can be enhanced by reducing inefficiencies, such as duplication and multiplication of the same information, and improved handling of medical information. The technology may lead to implanted, wearable, portable, or environmental implementations of stored information. Particularly, with increased deployment of hand-held and wireless devices, patient information can be kept in or accessed using these devices. The devices could become highly personalized, or health-aware, and may provide match on facilities nearby with the needs of the patient.

1.9.3 Patient-managed and Influenced Health

Many patients are uncomfortable or even paranoid of the use of technologies in their immediate environment. Also, in some cases, especially when patients are very old or have severe mental or physical limitations, patient involvement may not be possible such as those in nursing homes. But in most cases, the patients should be made more aware on how different technologies can improve their quality of life, especially those living alone in homes or assisted living facilities. Patients should be more involved in the technologies in the monitoring and preventive care. The technologies should be more intuitive to use and should be customized to the physical and mental abilities of the patients. During the customization, patient's input should be considered and valued. The technologies and components should be reliable, reusable, and should cause no harm to patients. On a more practical basis, if some patients are not able to participate in technology-enabled healthcare, the healthcare system should still be able to accommodate them in receiving care, which may be somewhat limited or more expensive.

By actively involving patients in the technology in, over and around them, it is expected that it will significantly improve the adherence with monitoring, treatment and medications. This will reduce the number of trips to emergency rooms, hospitalizations, and charges for healthcare professionals. Therefore, it will reduce the overall cost of healthcare services in the long-run. Certainly, technologies can expand the coverage and improve the delivery of healthcare services while utilizing the limited human resources more effectively, more research is needed in evaluating the impact of technologies in the overall "healing" and the long-term health of patients with or without much physical contact with healthcare professionals.

1.9.4 Active Role of Healthcare Professionals

Many times healthcare professionals are not very comfortable with the use of technologies as they fear that this could impact their work practices, lead to increased professional vulnerability, and lead to more cognitive load possibly resulting in additional medical errors. Although, some proven technologies have found their ways in the healthcare systems in reducing some inefficiencies related to administration and care. The healthcare professionals should be encouraged, or even convinced, to view technologies as a way to reduce medical errors, improve various processed, and reduce future costs. There should be more active role for healthcare professionals in using and managing technologies in healthcare. This could include use of best practices, support for security and privacy, and usability and preferences of healthcare professionals. It is also likely that the roles of healthcare professionals will evolve with technological evolution of healthcare system, more work is also needed in addressing the re-training needs of existing healthcare professionals as well as the training of future healthcare professionals.

1.9.5 More Efficient Delivery of Healthcare Services

The overall quality of healthcare, including pre- and post-hospitalization care, can be improved by many different ways. One is to provide patient-centric and patient-influenced care, where various rules and regulations evolve to focus on patient's needs. This will also require an increased involvement of patients and more informed patients. Another is to use health monitoring, where patients vital signs (BP, pulse, temperature, oxygen saturation in blood) and other biomedical parameters are monitored and recorded. A healthcare professional is alerted if one or more "abnormal" conditions arise. The use of monitoring will allow patients to be in different locations and intervention by healthcare professionals only when necessary. Finally, more efforts can be made to achieve more "personalized" healthcare.

1.10 Rest of the Book

The rest of the book is divided into eleven chapters and can be described as follows:

In chapter 2, we show how Information Technologies can play a major role in how healthcare services are designed, offered and utilized. More specifically, the topics of health informatics, electronic health, electronic health records, and telemedicine are discussed. Also, HIPAA is discussed in the context of IT and healthcare. Several challenges in the wide-scale deployment of electronic records are also presented. Many research problems are also identified and discussed.

In chapter 3, we first discuss current and emerging trends in pervasive computing including wearable computing and then present how pervasive computing can lead to pervasive healthcare. More specifically, examples of pervasive health monitoring, mobile telemedicine, intelligent emergency management service, health aware mobile device, pervasive access to health information, pervasive life style management, and medical inventory management system are presented.

Wireless networks form an important component of patient monitoring. In chapter 4, several networking requirements of wireless patient monitoring are identified, characteristics of wireless networks are presented, and how wireless networks can be used in health monitoring is also shown. More specifically, location management, reliability and bandwidth requirements are discussed. Traffic management in wireless networks for health monitoring is also included.

Health monitoring involves obtaining, processing, and analyzing vital signs and related parameters. In chapter 5, we discuss how these can be obtained and what specific vital signs can be used in detecting certain conditions. Several examples are presented, including monitoring of sleep apnea, arrhythmias, stress, and a range of mental illnesses. We conclude the chapter by identifying several possible monitoring types for future work including behavioral, sleep patterns, and eating patterns.

Wireless health monitoring can monitor patient's health anywhere anytime without affecting their daily lifestyle and use limited time of healthcare professionals more effectively. In chapter 6, we discuss the current work in wireless monitoring in six different categories, the evolution of patient monitoring, a framework and implementation of wireless patient monitoring system.

In wireless health monitoring, healthcare professionals will make decisions based on the knowledge derived from multiple set of informational items such as patient's medical history, current vital signs, medical knowledge, and specific patient conditions. In chapter 7, we discuss medical decision making by focusing on devices of healthcare professionals, requirements and functions of healthcare professionals, what to do when something goes wrong, and, how to manage cognitive load. Finally, how the medical decisions may be made in the future is presented.

There is considerable interest in using wireless and mobile technologies in patient monitoring in diverse environments including hospitals and nursing homes. In chapter 8, we discuss how infrastructure-oriented wireless networks, including commercial cellular/3G and versions of IEEE 802.11 wireless LANs, can be used to support health monitoring in diverse environments. Many related challenges are also addressed.

In some cases where coverage of infrastructure-oriented wireless networks is not available or reliable, ad hoc wireless networks can be used to support health monitoring. Chapter 9 focuses on how ad hoc networks can be used in wireless patient monitoring. The use of ad hoc networks does introduce several challenges including reliability, power management and routing. These challenges are discussed and several solutions are proposed.

Recently, health monitoring using ad hoc wireless networks has been proposed. Although innovative, such ad hoc networks primarily rely on the co-operation of devices and a lack of co-operation negatively affects the delivery of messages carrying patients' vital signs. In chapter 10, we discuss how reliable wireless health monitoring can be achieved using ad hoc networks, ways to obtain the cooperation of routing devices, and an incentive-based mechanism to improve wireless patient monitoring. The design of network protocols is also presented for decision making.

Context information in health monitoring can be used to improve the quality of healthcare delivery, utilize the limited healthcare and human resources more efficiently, and to move towards matching the healthcare services to the current medical conditions and needs of the patients under health monitoring. In chapter 11, we show how context-awareness can help healthcare services. More specifically, we address how the context may be generated and utilized in health monitoring. The evolution from context-awareness to health-awareness is also presented along with how more work can be done to address the current problems in context-awareness. Just like physical illnesses, people with mental illnesses can be treated and monitored for a range of conditions and provided medical care as necessary. In chapter 12, a new field of wireless psychiatry, or a way to address many problems using wireless technologies, is introduced. This includes comprehensive monitoring of patients for symptoms, behavior, and medication compliance. The monitoring includes suicidal and homicidal behavior, medication compliance, and related physical conditions such as sleep patterns and changes in weight. Several examples of mental health monitoring, medication compliance monitoring and disability monitoring are also presented.

Questions

1. List three different ways to reduce/slow the growth of US healthcare expenses.
2. Think of one unique way to reduce healthcare expenses. Describe this in more details on what would be needed and how will it work.
3. Discuss how technologies may help addressing the shortage of healthcare professionals?
4. Discuss three factors that may affect the adoption of the emerging technologies in healthcare.
5. Can preventive care reduce the cost of healthcare in short-term? What about long-term?
6. What are chronic diseases? Take a chronic disease and discuss how to manage it well to improve the quality of life for patients while reducing healthcare expenses.
7. Present your own possible evolution of healthcare system. Discuss why you think that it is likely to happen?
8. Discuss single-payer and multi-payers model for healthcare system. Are their any unique advantages of each of these two systems?

References
[1] Website   for   World   Health   Organization:
     http://www.who.int/whosis/database/core/core_select_process.cfm?strISO3_se-
     lect=ALL&strIndicator_select=nha&intYear_select=latest&fixed=indicator&language=engl
     ish
[2] U.S. Census Bureau (August 2007) Income, Poverty, and Health Insurance Coverage in the
     United States: 2006. (available at http://www.census.gov/prod/2007pubs/p60-233.pdf)
[3] Website   for   National   Healthcare   Expenditure   Data:
     http://www.cms.hhs.gov/NationalHealthExpendData/Downloads/proj2007.pdf

[4] US   Healthcare   Cost:
     http://www.kaiseredu.org/topics_im.asp?imID=1&parentID=61&id=358
[5] Wikipedia   on   US   Healthcare
     http://en.wikipedia.org/wiki/Health_care_in_the_United_States
[6] US Department of Health and Human Services, National Center for Health Workforce
     Analysis: U.S.   Health   Workforce   Personnel   Factbook   (available   at
     http://bhpr.hrsa.gov/healthworkforce/reports/factbook.htm)
[7] Source for population data: http://quickfacts.census.gov/qfd/states/00000.html
[8] US Department of Labor, Bureau of Labor Statistics: Occupational Outlook Handbook,
     2008-09 (available at http://www.bls.gov/oco/ocos074.htm)
[9] Emergency Department Visits by Persons Recently Discharged from U.S. Hospitals, July
     24, 2008.Center for Disease Control: National Health Statistics Reports (NHSR) (available
     at http://www.cdc.gov/nchs/data/nhsr/nhsr006.pdf)
[10] Nation's health dollar - where it came from, where it went (available at
     http://www.cms.hhs.gov/NationalHealthExpendData/downloads/PieChartSourcesExpenditu
     res2006.pdf)
[11] Makeham M, Dovey S, County M, Kidd M (2002) An international taxonomy for errors in
     general practice: a pilot study. Medical Journal of Australia, 177: 68-72, July 15th
[12] Thorpe K, Howard D (2006) The rise in spending among Medicare beneficiaries: the role of
     chronic disease prevalence and changes in treatment intensity. Health Affairs, 25(5): 378-
     388
[13] CDC Report (2007) Obesity among adults in the united states--no statistically significant
     change   since   2003-2004   (available   at
     http://www.cdc.gov/nchs/pressroom/07newsreleases/obesity.htm)
[14] US Institute of Medicine Report "To Err Is Human: Building a Safer Health System"
     (http://www.nap.edu/books/0309068371/html/)

Chapter 2: E-Health and IT in Healthcare

Abstract Information Technologies can play a major role in how healthcare services are designed, offered and utilized. In this chapter, we show how IT can be utilized in healthcare. More specifically, the topics of health informatics, electronic health, electronic health records, and telemedicine are discussed. Also, HIPAA is discussed in the context of IT and healthcare. Detailed discussion on medical records and several challenges in the wide-scale deployment are also presented. The future of telemedicine is also addressed.

2.1 E-health

E-health can be broadly defined as the application of information and communication technologies across the entire range of functions involved in the practice and delivery of healthcare. This could include a range of information such as patient's medical records (EMR), billing and payment information, employees and hospital information. One of the implementations of E-health today involves the use of the Internet for storing, accessing, and modifying healthcare information. However, e-health is a much broader field covering digitization of many healthcare processes and tasks, resulting in new names such as e-billing, e-payment, e-prescription, e-supply, and e-records.

The major thrusts behind the introduction and deployment of e-health are to obtain efficiencies in healthcare delivery and management, improvement in the quality of healthcare, cost reduction, reduction in medical errors, and moving healthcare resources to the place of needs. A simple architecture for e-health is shown in Figure 2.1 along with players that will have a major role in the future of e-health. Not all of the players will be involved in all facets of e-health, but will focus on digitization of their processes and facilitate the use of these processes by others. For example, pharmacies will be focusing on e-prescriptions and e-refills and will facilitate doctors and other healthcare professionals to be able to access and place their orders for various medications. The insurance companies will focus on e-billing and e-payments to healthcare and service providers such as hospitals, doctors, and pharmacies. The regulators will ensure certain quality of care by accessing a range of information including e-records. This could be the part of e-audit application. The patients may not have complete access to all information, but will be informed of results, diagnosis, prescriptions, appointments, insurance and related information. The patient's request for additional information will be processed and results will be relayed to the patient or his/her designated agent.

U. Varshney, *Pervasive Healthcare Computing: EMR/EHR, Wireless and Health Monitoring*,   17
DOI: 10.1007/978-1-4419-0215-3_2,
© Springer Science + Business Media, LLC 2009

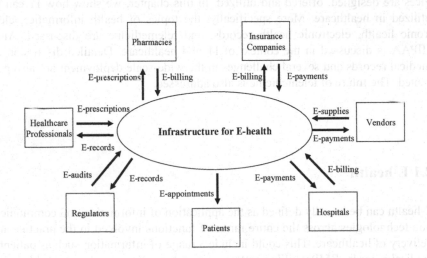

Fig. 2.1 Major Players and Applications in E-health

Another emerging area of serious interest is Health Informatics. Health Informatics or medical informatics is the intersection of several fields including information science, computer science, healthcare, and business. Health Informatics deals with the resources, devices, and, methods required for optimizing the acquisition, storage, retrieval, and use of information in health and biomedicine [2]. Using this broad definition, HI could have several components including (a) electronic medical records, (b) decision support systems for healthcare, (c) health information systems, (d) protocols for exchange of medical and healthcare information, and, (e) devices for medical decisions.

The coverage and relationship among various terms in this chapter are shown in Figure 2.2. E-health is broader than health informatics as it also includes the delivery of actual care, while the latter focuses only on how a range of information is utilized in various healthcare processes. Similarly, both telemedicine and m-health have technological as well as delivery of healthcare functions. There has been a lot of progress in each of these areas and will be covered with more details. More specifically, medical records and telemedicine are covered in the next few sections.

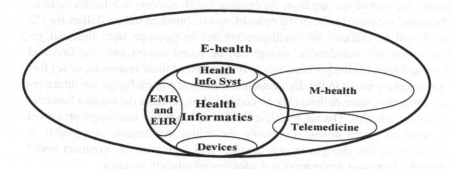

Fig. 2.2 The Relationship and Coverage of E-health and Health Informatics

2.1.1 Challenges in E-health

There are several challenges and obstacles that must be addressed before e-health becomes prevalent. These challenges primarily deal with how the medical and healthcare information has been collected and stored, lack of technologies and potential cost to digitize the existing processes and tasks. To start with, most of the existing medical and healthcare information is present in multiple formats including paper-based records. Converting all of it to electronic format is a major challenge with some of the handwritten information as physician notes. The use of a standard form to collect information from patients may be helpful for conversion to digital format. There are also challenges of potential disruption in the care, significant load and learning for healthcare professionals, and lack of incentives in some cases.

Even as some of the information is being digitized and converted to electronic domain, it is observed that several different systems of e-health are evolving. Some of these are closed or non-standardized proprietary systems, which do not support interoperability with other systems thus resulting in islands of e-health that are difficult to interconnect. The use of an interoperability certification could solve most of the interoperability problems.

The current healthcare systems have introduced a range of technologies in very ad hoc fashion and have not kept with shifts in technological evolution for several reasons, including the cost, complexity and rate of technological changes. These factors prevent the existing healthcare systems from utilizing many benefits of the current and emerging information and communications technologies. To address these, most promising technologies should be identified and thoroughly evaluated for their suitability to healthcare systems.

Certainly, the cost of moving from the existing health systems to e-health systems is substantial, estimated to be of the order of several hundred billion dollars for US alone. It will be difficult for healthcare entities to generate such financial resources unless (a) considerable savings can be found somewhere else first and then applied here, (b) the governments provide some of these resources, or (c) for-profit companies invest in the digitization of healthcare in exchange for future returns. In practice, these options may be combined to generate the needed financial resources for e-health. The achievable efficiencies in various healthcare processes could result in future savings exceeding the initial investments in e-health. It should be noted that changes in organizations and regulatory environment could also help the increased deployment and adoption of e-health systems.

2.1.2 Privacy and Security in E-health

Privacy relates to private information and people's ability to have some control over their private information. Security relates with the ability to keep information secure from unintended recipients. Taken together, privacy and security are big challenges due to potential threats to sensitive healthcare data and abuse of health-care benefits.

Regulatory frameworks such as HIPAA (Health Insurance Portability and Accountability Act of 1996) have been designed to limit the use of what medical information can be transmitted, stored, displayed, and utilized [1]. All healthcare systems in US must be HIPAA compliant. HIPAA defines Protected Health Information (PHI), which includes individually identifiable health information related to the past, present and future physical and mental health conditions and payments for healthcare services. HIPAA provides a set of standard policies for healthcare providers to protect a patient's privacy. It also provides a standard set of electronic transactions formats and regulations to ensure the privacy and security of healthcare related transactions. The 4 standards or rules are Privacy, Security, Identifiers, and Transactions and Code Sets. HIPAA provides several rights for patients. More specifically, there are six patient-rights in HIPAA [1]:

1. The right to inspect/get a copy of own medical records
2. The right to request the correction of inaccurate health information
3. The right to find out where PHI has been shared for purposes other than care, payment, or healthcare operations
4. The right to request special restrictions on the use or disclosure of PHI
5. The right to request PHI to be shared with the patient in a particular way (home address/office address etc.)
6. The right to file complaints (if any is violated)

HIPAA requires that all covered entities (such as hospitals) appoint a privacy officer, develop proper privacy procedures, and implement access control for all stored media. HIPAA was originally proposed for reducing "insurance-related health transactions" cost, but has evolved to become a major framework for ensuring privacy in healthcare services. However, the overhead of HIPAA compliance is likely to increase the cost for healthcare providers, insurers, health plan providers and claims clearing houses, which process claims on behalf of healthcare providers. Also, the complexity faced by patients in finding out who may have had access to their PHI or getting incorrect information fixed is currently quite significant. There are many instances of privacy where either HIPAA is not applicable or effective, and in some cases it is cumbersome to be fully compliant. Certainly, work is needed in extending the range of HIPAA to include more covered entities already dealing with healthcare information, while simplifying its compliance.

In paper-based healthcare, vulnerabilities were limited to the site where such files were kept in the shelf. However, in e-health environment, patient information may be stored on one or more servers over a network, which may be vulnerable to attacks from hackers and thieves; and human mistakes such as misplacing laptops and other devices with patient information. Some networks are known for good end-to-end security, however, in practice, there are varying levels of security in networks. Additionally, some networks, especially wireless LANs, are vulnerable to hackers with analysis of packets. There have been many improvements, but the end-to-end security is still a problem. With these challenges, there is some concern in the healthcare community about identity theft leading to misuse of healthcare benefits. In many cases, the privacy and security are cited as the major obstacles in e-health by hospital administrators.

HIPAA will affect e-health and future healthcare delivery in more than one ways. This will include who can access and modify EMR, who can see what is displayed on a screen in a hospital, the use of mobile and wireless devices, processes in emergency care, telemedicine, and healthcare delivery in an assisted living and in nursing homes. This will require that only certain healthcare professionals could access EMR, computers and devices in care of patients have restricted access, information is encrypted before transmission over networks, and only certain healthcare professionals and caregivers can receive notifications on patient's conditions on their mobile devices. If the PHI is transmitted over a network, the network packets should not be logged or read by anyone else managing the network infrastructure. Also, if a mobile or handheld device is used by some one other than designated healthcare professionals, it should not have any stored information that could be considered as PHI.

For the end-to-end HIPAA compliance, IT-enabled systems of each healthcare entity must be HIPAA compliant when operating in isolation as well as when interoperating with systems of other entities. The use of emerging technologies in implanted, wearable, portable and environmental implementations for healthcare must be ensured for HIPAA compliance for their wide-scale use in healthcare processes and delivery.

2.2 EMR and EHR

Electronic medical records (EMRs) are digital representation of patient's health-care information including identification, lab tests, diagnostic tests, medications and physician notes. One of the biggest challenges in healthcare is both the number of sources where the data may come from and the sheer amount of data that is generated. Not all of this data is relevant for a given condition or treatment, and therefore deciding what is relevant and what is not is also a challenge. EMR is an attempt to put together most relevant set of data needed in the patient care. Therefore, it normally includes patient's history, various tests and medications, and billing information. A complete EMR system from a vendor would include EMR software and applications, EMR hardware, installation, training and support.

In common usage, EMR and EHR (Electronic Health Record) have been used interchangeably, but these are two different things. An EMR is a legal record created in hospitals and ambulatory environments, while EHR represents the ability to easily share medical information such as EMRs among various healthcare stakeholders and to have a patient's information follow him or her. The healthcare stakeholders could include patients/consumers, healthcare providers, employers, payers, and insurers including the state and federal governments. In cases of potential bio-warfare and epidemics, many state and federal security agencies may have serious interest in medical records of populations in certain regions. One example may be to look at medication patterns for patients in a certain region to locate the source of epidemic or spreading of diseases.

2.2.1 Advantages of EMR

As an interesting insight, compared to paper-based records, EMRs can be used by multiple users simultaneously, are available 24x7 to close-by and remote locations, and are always legible [3]. The availability of EMR avoids the patient having to fill up several pages of medical history and current treatment, potentially with errors of recollection and haste. Although involving significant initial cost, EMR has been shown to be effective in medical decision making and could cut the cost of healthcare in the long-run. EMR has also been shown to reduce the length of stay in hospitals, decrease adverse drug events, improve continuity of care, and reduce practice variations [3]. These benefits are realized as the most relevant information is readily available in the medical records for effective decision making, detection of possible interactions of medications, and subsequent and more standardized care of the patient. The number of medical errors could also be reduced as handwritten notes and prescriptions do not have to be interpreted as in the older paper-based records.

2.2.2 EMR Adoption

Worldwide, the usage is much higher, such as Netherlands and New Zealand with 90% or higher rates, however, the adoption rate in US has been slow. According to a recent survey, only 4% of US physicians have access to fully functional electronic health records and only 13% have access to basic electronic records [4]. Out of the physicians using these records, 97% to 99% have been using most or all the functions. For larger practices with 50 or more physicians, the similar adoption rate jumps to 17 and 33% [4]. Among the adopters, the advantages cited include improved quality of medical decisions, better communications, faster prescription refills, timely access to information, and reduction in medical errors. Financial factors were ranked as the biggest barrier to the adoption [4], thus smaller and individual practices showed significantly lower adoption rates. Additionally, there are some other reasons behind this low level of adoption in US. As the US does not have a nationalized healthcare, unlike most western countries, and most care is provided by a large number of private medical groups and hospitals. Many of these facilities, especially smaller ones, are very cost-sensitive and many physicians perceive EMR as a step against their autonomy. Even within US, where care is provided by single entity, the adoption rates are high. A major example is Department of Veteran's Affair (VA), which deals with healthcare for people that are serving/have served in armed forces, in US has an EMR system which can be accessed at its more than one thousand healthcare facilities.

Within US, there are several mandates in place to encourage the use of electronic records, such as US government's EHR 2014, which requires national EHR capability by 2014, less than five years from now. As part of this mandate, the government has created an Office of the National Coordinator (ONC) for Health Information Technology within the department of Health and Human Services [12]. The ONC coordinates the efforts of the department towards development of standards and implementation of a nationwide health IT infrastructure for achieving the goal of EHR 2014. The HHS is also distributing some grants to encourage health IT projects and is also involved in evaluating the effectiveness of EHR initiatives. The total cost has been estimated to exceed $100 billion for nationwide EHR in US. However, spread over several years, it only represents an increase of a few percent to the total healthcare expenses.

2.2.3 PHR Support by Private Companies

In a related development, some companies in US are also offering storage for health information, termed as Personal Health Records (PHRs). Here, the patients are asked to create and update their own health records on certain protected websites. Two such examples are Google Health and HealthVault by Microsoft.

In Google Health, patients are asked to create health profiles using their known conditions; import medical records form hospitals, labs and pharmacies; find information on their conditions; fill their prescription online; and allow their choice of healthcare facilities to import the health information [5]. There are several advantages of such system. It encourages and empowers patients to create health profile and put all healthcare information together. The ability to search for related (and not all) information on a certain condition is also helpful. But there could also be some limitations. The first, most patients lack the knowledge to interpret or analyze their medical records and may come up with incorrect and even dangerous interpretations. The entered information may not be the most accurate or complete as it is the patient's view of his/her health information. In general, the trained healthcare professionals are both more qualified and objective as far as dealing with healthcare information is concerned.

In HealthVault [6], patients can save their healthcare information and also share it with people they trust such as family members and friends. It also allows them to create a document with list of medical conditions, medications, and healthcare providers that can be used in emergencies by family members and friends. Some patients may be uncomfortable with who can access their online information and their lack of technical knowledge needed in some specific interactions with online systems.

Although these attempts should be lauded for their service to the society as well as indirectly pressuring the healthcare entities to put their EMR/EHR systems together quickly, more efforts are needed to ensure that healthcare information is not deleted, modified, and/or accessed by someone else and thus remains reliably usable in cases of emergencies. Some automated system may also be needed to generate warnings for conflicts, created by information entered by the patient. If the patients have not added/updated all information or have not imported all medical information form one or more sources, the usefulness of such services may be limited. However, on the other side, such PHR can lead to lifelong medical records for patients and allow for continued care in case of patients moving to locations where their EMR/EHR can not be accessed.

2.2.4 EMR Architecture

There are many definitions and interpretation of what constitutes an EMR. We consider an EMR to include sections for patient information and history, orders for prescriptions, orders for tests, reporting of test results, billing information and physician notes. There may also be sections for recent drug advisory and any unusual medical conditions. The structure of EMR along with possible interactions with physicians and laboratories are shown in Figure 2.3. Certainly, there are restrictions on who can access the EMR and these restrictions may be enforced to achieve compliance to HIPAA. In simple terms, the healthcare professionals directly involved in the care of the patient may be able to access and modify EMR. The information could be displayed to a physician or a healthcare professional in a certain way, which may have been customized before to suit the type of healthcare facility and the preferences of healthcare professionals. The patient information may come from multiple sources including patient himself/herself and older paper-based records. This process may be simplified by using standardized forms and/or involving the patient in entering and verifying the patient information. The physician may order for lab tests and may write some notes. Later the requests for tests are fulfilled by a laboratory and test results are posted. Then the physician may be informed and he/she makes a diagnosis and may order for medications, which is sent to designated pharmacy after checking for any possible interactions with existing medications. The pharmacy may also check for any such problems. Once the pharmacy fills the order, EMR is updated to show that the medication has been dispensed.

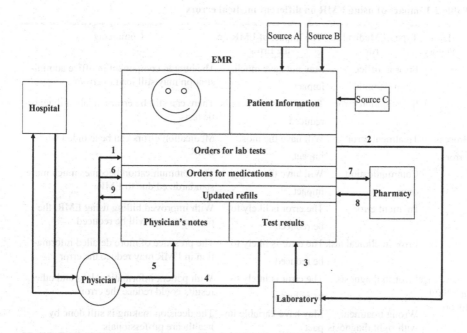

Fig. 2.3 Basic Architecture and Interactions of an Electronic Medical Record

2.2.5 Reduction of Medical Errors with EMR

One of the major reasons behind EMR adoption is to reduce the number of medical errors. As there are several different types of medical errors, it may be interesting to discuss which ones will be reduced more than the others. We use the error classification developed for general practice [8]. The types of medical errors are broken into two major categories: process errors and knowledge/skill errors. As there are a large number of errors, only the most common errors are included in the Table 2.1. For each error, the possible impact of EMR is included and relevant information is presented as comments. More specifically, if the error is "wrong treatment with right diagnosis", the impact of EMR is variable depending on the condition and the treatment. Some of the types of wrong treatments can be easily flagged by intelligent EMRs, some by the patient, some by pharmacist and some by insurance companies at a later date. Some more complex treatment errors could be missed and that is why the impact of EMR is variable on such errors.

Table 2.1 Impact of using EMR on different medical errors

Major Category	Type of Medical Error	The Impact of EMR on the Error	Comments
	Error in office administration	May not have much impact	The human component in office administration may still lead to errors
	Investigation error	The error is likely to be reduced	There can still be errors in lab or diagnostic tests
Process Errors	Treatment error	Will have the most impact	Medication errors can be avoided with EMR
	Communication error	Will have the most impact	The communication becomes much more standardized due to EMR
	Payment error	The error is likely to be reduced	With improved billing using EMR, the payment error will be reduced
	Error in clinical task	The error is likely to be reduced	The presence of more detailed information in EMR may reduce the error
Knowledge and Skill Errors	Error in diagnosis	The error is likely to be reduced	With patient information, labs and other results could reduce the error
	Wrong treatment with right diagnosis	May have variable impact	The decision making is still done by healthcare professionals

2.2.6 Achieving EHR Functionality

The national Electronic Health Record functionality can be created in several different ways. This includes creating local databases of EMRs at a healthcare entity involved in providing the initial care to the patients. The EMRs can then be requested by other healthcare facilities with network access. The other way to facilitate EHR may be to create multiple national databases of EMRs, which can be accessed directly without going through the facility that created them in the first place (Figure 2.4). Both of these options have some limitations. First, creating national databases of EMRs is an enormous task. Any local update in EMR should also be made in the EMR in the national databases. Providing secure access to authorized personnel to so many different possible records is another challenge. If it can not be created for all patients, then national databases could be created for specific conditions such as cancers, mental disorders, diabetes, strokes, and pulmonary illnesses. Such a system would be a wonderful asset for both treatment and research in specific illnesses. For example, EMRs for patients with depression treated nationwide can be kept in one database to support better outcome studies comparing morbidity and mortality region-wide and nationwide, and also to compare treatment outcomes in different regions of the country. Storing EMRs locally may be easier, but the requesting healthcare facility must have to know where the EMRs are stored and that site should be available for such access.

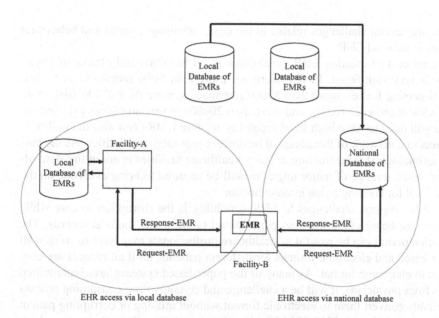

Fig. 2.4 Two Ways to Achieve National EHR Functionality: Local and National Access

One possible way to implement US wide National Health Information Network is by creating and connecting Regional Health Information Organizations. These organizations bring together all stake holders in a well defined geographical area and facilitate information exchange among them [11].

Once national EHR capability is achieved, more efforts would be needed to create international EHR to provide medical information across countries. Such facility would be required when someone from one country goes to another and needs medical treatment, while all his/her medical information is in his/her country of residence. The international EHR may be implemented by co-ordination among individual national databases. Recently, a group of 11 EU countries announced the work on creating an EHR capability across these countries.

2.3 Issues in EMR/EHR

2.3.1 The Major Challenges to National EHR

There are several challenges related to the cost, technology, social and behavioral factors in national EHR.

The total cost of creating EHR capabilities in all hospitals and offices of physicians is very significant. In US, there are more than 5000 hospitals, more than 19000 nursing homes, more than 59000 pharmacies, more than 63000 labs, more than 4800 emergency rooms, and more than 200000 physician offices [3]. Each of these will need to have both local capability to store EMRs and also the ability to connect to a network of thousands of healthcare providers and entities. As the current technological infrastructure at many healthcare facilities is not at the state-of-the-art level, a range of major upgrades will be required to bring everyone on the same level for creating a rich interconnection.

One of the biggest challenges to EHR capability is the disruption to care while systems are being upgraded from paper-based to electronic medical records. The transition period can be painful as healthcare professionals may have to work with paper-based and electronic formats for different patients, until all records are converted to electronic format. As many of the paper-based systems have handwritten notes from physicians, it will be a challenge and certainly time-consuming process to reliably convert them to electronic format without missing or corrupting patient information. Although EHR 2014 is only a few years away, these factors are slowing down the level of progress needed to meet the EHR mandated deadline.

The interoperability between different electronic systems in terms of formats, messages, and representations will be a major challenge. There are more than 25 different formats of EMR today in US alone and many of which may not fully inter-operate with one another. Additionally, the performance of these EMR systems could vary from 99% availability (less than 1% downtime) to no such performance guarantee. It should be noted that performance degradation of EMR systems could affect critical care. In some cases, EMR systems have to be customized to individual practices with unique requirements such as those of multi-specialty, multi-location facilities. The customization may make the interoperability even more difficult to achieve. The good news is that there is a standardization body called Certification Commission on Healthcare Information Technology (CCHIT) [9], which is working with vendors to certify EMR systems. The solution to these interoperability problems is to design and implement a common or universal format. There are several standards to facilitate a range of medical communications. The primary one is HL7 (health level 7), which facilitate exchange of healthcare information [10]. DICOM is another messaging standard primarily used with radiographic images.

The privacy and legal aspects also add more challenges to EHR. Many patients are uncomfortable with the sheer number of people with access to their medical information even with many restrictions from HIPAA. With national EHR, even more people may have access to the patient information. Further, networks and infrastructure may be vulnerable to hackers who may want to access EHR records of certain people. But as no system is going to be perfect, these may do much more good to the patient, while potentially causing some harm in some isolated cases.

There are organizational challenges as many healthcare professionals are not convinced that national EHR would improve the quality or delivery of healthcare. Many of them are against it and feel that it may impact their work habits. Some physicians believe that their productivity may be reduced, especially in the short-term. Some are also concerned about the increased access and peer-review to their work and potential for increased lawsuit and claims. However, this will certainly improve the quality of care from some healthcare professionals.

There are several technological challenges to national EHR. In general, there are limitations in what hardware, software and networks can do, the reliability and security of infrastructure is not guaranteed, and the cost of upgrades and repairs may be high. Sometimes infrastructure can not meet the stringent medical requirements without a high degree of redundancy, thus increasing the cost significantly. The technologies become obsolete in short period of time, thus requiring the move to another set of technologies and adding to the cost of doing business with additional training. Many times the EMR vendors may not provide the adequate IT support for their systems or may discontinue the products in preference to newer products. As the patients could ask for old records as part of HIPAA rights, very reliable and long-term backups of patient information will be required. This will add to the total cost of EMR/EHR.

2.3.2 Access to EMR/EHR

With HIPAA and other regulation, only authorized people should be allowed to access EMR. This could include all the people involved in the care of the patient currently such as the physician, nurse and the specialist. The EHR systems can utilize context information in deciding who may need to access medical records and the level of access such as read only, or read and modify certain information. To provide security, encryption and digital signatures can be utilized on stored information and access to the information. There has been some work in addressing security in healthcare environment. In one such work, the use of XML cryptographic techniques including encryption and signature has been shown to provide a level of security against malicious users especially when used in conjunction with role based authorization [14]. Another study evaluated several options for providing secure access to patient records including 802.11i and IPsec (IP security protocol) [15]. The authors found that this additional layer of security allows for secure authentication and authorization, secure communications and also maintains integrity of the information [15].

To address many privacy concerns, the access to EMR could be logged to show who accessed it for how long, what information was read, and what if any changes were made. Such features would lead to more effective restriction on sensitive healthcare information. The access logs can also be used to improve the future access to EMR and healthcare information.

2.3.3 Use of Handheld Devices to Access EMR

With increasing deployment of handheld and wireless devices, healthcare professionals will need to access medical records using these devices with limited screen size. As the entire records may be difficult to display for proper viewing, the system could display only the requested/needed components and allow the navigation through the record as needed. If the entire record must be viewed for medical decisions, the system may display the whole record on a nearby larger screen to the authorized healthcare professionals. There should also be some restrictions on healthcare professionals using their personal mobile devices for accessing EMRs.

There has been some work in developing mobile frontends to EMR/EHR systems including MARiS [13]. The authors reported that they observed various healthcare processes and designed the interface to mimic the existing procedures including actual process structure, terminology, familiar visual elements and symbols [13]. Since users were actively involved in the development of actual tool, user acceptance was easier to obtain [13]. The future work will involve moving away from the existing processes to the ones that could exploit the enhanced capabilities of computers. The authors also reported that MARiS contributed to an increased quality of medical treatment and volume of billed treatments resulted in financial payoffs in about one year [13].

In an environment where patient data may be distributed and fragmented, it is difficult to integrate and present to healthcare professionals for effective decision making. One solution to this problem is addressed in MobileMed [18]. More specifically, the existing health systems send the patient data in HL7 messages to a central database, which integrates all patient information and makes them accessible to mobile devices via a web server [18].

With emerging technologies such as computing grids and mobile devices, it may be possible to employ streaming as a way to send information to healthcare professionals in addition to just faster downloads. This is even more applicable for images that are obtained from multiple diagnostic devices. One such work focuses on using these technologies to support streaming-based access to image and data management functions [19]. The authors have also shown that there is positive impact on clinical workflows.

2.3.4 Access to EMR in Emergency

In emergency cases, the patient may not be able to provide any identifying information to a healthcare professional for EHR access. This would be ironic as the main purpose of such access would be to help the patient when most needed. There are several possible ways to address this. One is to store the identifying information on an RFID (radio frequency identification) chip, which can either be implanted in the patient or more likely kept as a wearable or portable item. When needed, the healthcare professionals could use RFID reader to obtain the necessary information. If this is not possible, then the system could allow some or partial access to EMR in emergencies even if the authorization is not completed as long as the context information include patient in an emergency room and receiving care from the healthcare professional. Another possibility is to provide access to EMR via person's cell phone as many emergency medical services utilize a person's cell phone for identification.

The access to EMR in emergency is really is a trade-off between privacy and benefits and the regulatory environment should allow such exceptions. The system may not allow modification to EMR, but could store changes in another part and once the authorization is completed later, allow the changes to be completed. Also, once the emergency is over, the system can switch back to the original level of security. Any released information during an emergency in the best interest of patient can be logged and analyzed later both for how the information was used and also for improving the processes of releasing information.

In Denmark, EMRs are accessible to physicians even if they are not involved in the care of the patient. A very high-level of interoperability among multiple systems also increases the probability that such information can be accessed. The philosophy used in Danish health systems is that no patient should die because the system blocked access to a vital data [7]. Any such access will show as a violation with a log of who accessed what information [7], but could be very helpful in cases of emergency where patient may not be able to provide information to access his/her EMR.

2.3.5 Potential for Errors in EMR/EHR

Although, EMR systems will eliminate or reduce medical errors, especially those dealing with lack of information including adverse drug events, it may still have some errors. There are several different ways where errors may be introduced in EMR systems. This could include errors when patient information was converted from paper to electronic form and some of the information may have been handwritten on the paper. Such errors could be checked as the part of reliable conversion from paper to electronic formats. The patient may be allowed to enter personal vital information about him/her self directly on EMR or at least allowed to verify authenticity of information.

Assuming there are no introduced errors due to format conversion or the EMR was created digitally without conversion, healthcare professionals may make errors in entering one or more of patient information. This could include the case when labs were ordered incorrectly or the lab results were entered incorrectly. These could lead to errors in EMR and as the errors can get propagated, where an error leads to one or more errors and so on, it becomes very difficult to detect errors and then correct these. Both human and automated checking for potential errors should be employed to avoid errors in EMR systems. Intelligent EMRs could be designed to avoid errors by a range of automated processing of entered and stored information on patients and using current healthcare knowledge.

2.3.6 Current Research and Development Work

There are many current and emerging research problems related to medical records. These in general deal with interoperability of different EMR systems using middleware and other enhancements, how the information can be presented to healthcare professionals in the best possible way, how to design life-long EMRs for patients, how to avoid identity thefts and identity confusion among patients, different and multiple ways to authenticate people for EMR access, how to increase EMR adoption rate, and how to deal with large amount of data.

Another challenging problem is to derive and utilize knowledge from EMRs. This could also include finding patterns from EMRs which may help in detecting spread of diseases and quality of care. It will be an interesting challenge to store, process, represent, and access a large amount of EMR data. Another angle to this problem may be to treat this as a knowledge management problem, where healthcare professionals make decisions based on knowledge that is presented. This knowledge is created from multiple set of informational items in EMRs, but more work is needed in knowledge presentation, knowledge distribution, and knowledge application. Knowledge application or use of knowledge in a particular context is an interesting challenge and will require some efforts from healthcare professionals.

The national EHR ability would significantly improve both the quality and coverage of healthcare services. The quality would improve as detailed and current information on the patient would become available where it is needed. The coverage would improve as people can receive healthcare services in far-away and isolated places where they may be traveling to. Once the technology challenges of interoperability, storage, access, and security are addressed, the national EHR would also cut down on unnecessary tests, procedures and treatments with the availability of much more detailed and current patient information. This could significantly reduce the healthcare cost, while improving the quality of healthcare services.

There are challenges in how to best represent the diverse set of medical data to healthcare professionals. The current representations primarily are text-centric, which are not necessarily the best representation from a cognitive point of view. There is some work in visualizing electronic medical records to assist physicians with clinical tasks and medical decision-making such as the TimeLine system [16]. This uses a temporal visualization for medical data as the information contained with medical records is re-organized around medical disease entities and conditions [16]. The automatic construction of the TimeLine display involves data access, data mapping and re-organization, and data visualization. This allows for quick and comprehensive communication of the information to healthcare professionals to allow improved decision making [16].

Another on-going research in EMR/EHR deals with how to provide life-long medical record for continued care as patients move from one place to the other. Such detailed records that are accessible from anywhere anytime will also assist in a range of medical decision making, clinical research and health policy. The use of web services in EMR has been suggested in [17], where service oriented architecture is utilized in creating a lifelong EMR.

2.4 Telemedicine

Telemedicine can be broadly defined as the use of telecommunications technologies to provide medical and healthcare services to patients over a distance. Telemedicine has been in use in several places for about thirty years. It is significantly much more complex than teleconferencing and telecommuting due to its own set of challenges. In telemedicine, the focus is on diagnosis and treatment of patients and in some cases, legal and regulatory challenges exist as obstacle for widespread deployment. One major issue is the quality of telemedicine patient care. There has been some work which shows that telemedicine can result in effective delivery of healthcare in many appropriate conditions.

Telemedicine is driven by the need to provide healthcare services to people who will not be able to travel due to health problems, are not allowed to travel such as those in jail, or are in places far way from specialists including those involved in accident needing pre-hospitalization care. In telemedicine, normally two or more locations are joined together by video monitoring systems and networks to allow physicians, healthcare personnel, and patients to interact (Figure 2.5). The information traveling between sites is also encrypted to be HIPAA compliant. Also, the discussion may involve using the help of a specialist who could not be in the same location as everyone else. In some cases, only physicians are involved to discuss problems, diagnosis, and treatment for patients without having patients physically present. Telemedicine can be either real-time interactive consults or asynchronous where request-response occur in non real-time.

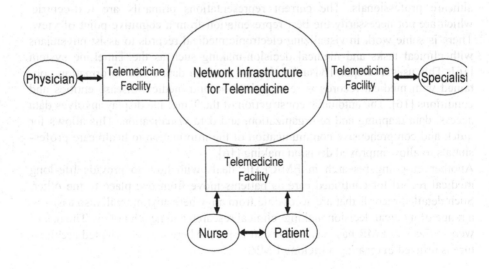

Fig. 2.5 A General Architecture of Telemedicine with Three Locations

2.4.1 Driving Forces behind Telemedicine

Telemedicine is generally used to cover large number of places including under-served, rural, communities; to utilize physicians in other locations including large cities; to expand practice base of physicians; to improve the quality of life for patients in nursing homes, homes, and hospitals; to reduce the cost of healthcare services; for improvement in the preventive care; and overall efficient utilization of healthcare resources. Many applications of telemedicine are preventive medicine especially in rural and underserved areas, counseling and tele-psychiatry, tele-radiology, assisted tele-surgery, consultation on lab-reports/tests, emergency and accidents. There have been telemedicine systems used in airplanes, cruise ships, and in emergency vehicles to provide necessary care for traveling patients.

One of the major applications of telemedicine is in trauma care, before the patient can be brought to a hospital. Such pre-hospital care has been addressed in [20], where a portable tele-trauma system supports the transmission of a patient's video, medical images, and electrocardiogram signals. This has been shown over a 3G commercial cellular network. The system in essence allows a trauma specialist to be virtually present at the remote location participate in the pre-hospital care [20]. The authors also present several enhancements, including media transformations, data prioritization, and application-level congestion to compensate for the limited and variable bandwidth of wireless links [20].

Another major area where telemedicine can have major impact is the management of chronic conditions. As the chronic diseases are major part of the healthcare expenses and are unlikely to be completely cured, it is important that these are managed well to reduce both the suffering of the patients as well as reducing the total cost of healthcare. One of the major chronic diseases is chronic obstructive pulmonary disease (COPD). A telemedicine system and related details for COPD is presented in [21]. The authors used two groups of patients in a clinical experiment and showed that fewer patients with access to telemedicine tools, such as access to call center and problem reporting, were readmitted [21].

2.4.2 Challenges for Telemedicine

Telemedicine has been experiencing a range of challenges. These include technical challenges such as suitability, usability, availability, maintainability, and upgradability. Each telemedicine system is designed to provide certain set of healthcare services and thus may not be suitable to other services. For example, a low resolution system designed for tele-psychiatry may not be suitable for cancer diagnosis involving complex radiographic images. Due to technical limitations, some of the telemedicine systems can not be upgraded to the changing requirement. The end-systems in telemedicine should be compatible to one another.

The major management challenges are the training of employees and adoption and use of technologies. The patient-centric and healthcare challenges include the quality of care, errors and potential harm. In practice, these challenges limit what a telemedicine system can do and how it is used. Another major challenge is the total cost. In practice, many telemedicine systems start from governmental grants to perform a specialized function, but after the grant expires the systems are not usable due to poor maintenance/lack of upgrade.

Telemedicine experience a range of regulatory restrictions, such as a physician not able to deliver care to patients in another state in US using telemedicine systems and the healthcare professionals receive lesser to no reimbursement for their telemedicine services.

2.4.3 The Future of Telemedicine

More work is needed in designing, implementing and deploying ubiquitous and mobile telemedicine systems, where physicians, healthcare providers and patients are no longer restricted to certain locations where telemedicine equipments are kept. This will be a major advance in telemedicine. The mobile telemedicine will allow the use of ever increasing mobile and wireless technologies, networks and devices. This will allow the coverage of telemedicine to reach to very remote places as long as some basic form of wireless connectivity exists. Certainly, more work is needed in analyzing the quality of telemedicine sessions with wireless technologies involving slower bit rates, small screen size, and privacy challenges. The work is needed on identifying specific telemedicine applications that could be supported by mobile and wireless infrastructure of varying degrees. One application could involve using SMS and text messaging as a way to support non-real-time to semi-real-time telemedicine functions.

2.5 Future of IT in Healthcare

E-health will change the way healthcare services are delivered, affecting all players involved in the delivery of healthcare to patients. As the paper-based systems are being converted to e-health systems using multiple different technologies, the interoperability of different e-health systems is becoming a major challenge. All e-health challenges should be addressed together including organizational where physicians need to be convinced that e-health can improve the quality of healthcare delivery without a loss of their autonomy. Also, the tasks and requirements should be derived first before technology should be selected. The cost issue is one of the most critical challenges. The governmental and private investment should be made along with incentives for higher payments for facilities with certain e-health infrastructure. Certainly, more work is needed on specific medical errors that can be reduced by e-health and return-on-investment for practices of different sizes, locations, and specialties.

Questions:
1. What is e-health and in what ways it can make the healthcare processes more efficient?
2. Which major healthcare player may benefit the most from e-health? Discuss your position.
3. What is health informatics and how it is different from e-health? Which one deals with information and which one deals with the delivery of healthcare also?
4. How do you see e-health, m-health, mobile devices, telemedicine, EMR/EHR, and health informatics fitting with one another? Draw a diagram to show any overlap.
5. Think of ways to create global Electronic Health Records. Draw a diagram and provide details.
6. What role do you see for PHR? Should someone rely more on EHR or PHR?
7. Discuss how medical errors could be reduced using EMR.
8. What role do you see for telemedicine in future healthcare?
9. Can it be said that telemedicine systems are precursor to emerging health monitoring systems? If you convert a telemedicine system to a health monitoring system, what loss of functionality would occur?
10. What is mobile telemedicine? What limitations must be overcome before mobile telemedicine could be widely deployed.
11. Find out more information on how telemedicine services are reimbursed? Also look at restrictions on providing telemedicine-based care in another state.

References
[1] Website for HIPAA: http://www.hhs.gov/ocr/hipaa
[2] Wikipedia: http://en.wikipedia.org/wiki/Medical_informatics
[3] Tierney W, Zafar A (2002) EMRs: An Introductory Tutorial, Available at http://healthit.ahrq.gov/portal/server.pt/gateway/PTARGS_0_251_0_0_18/EMR%20Talk.ppt
[4] DesRoches C et.al (2008) Electronic Health Records in Ambulatory Care-A National Survey of Physicians. New England Journal of Medicine, 359(1):50-60, July 3
[5] Website for Google Health: http://www.google.com/health
[6] Website for HealthVault: http://www.healthvault.com
[7] Moller J, Vosegaard H (2008) Experiences with electronic health records. IEEE IT Professional, 10(2): 19-23, March-April
[8] Makeham M, Dovey S, County M, Kidd M (2002) An international taxonomy for errors in general practice: a pilot study. Medical Journal of Australia, 177: 68-72, July 15th
[9] Website for CCHIT: http://www.cchit.org
[10] Website for Hl7: http://www.HL7.org

[11] Wikipedia for Regional Health Information Organizations at http://en.wikipedia.org/wiki/RHIO

[12] Website for Office of National Coordinator for HIT: http://www.hhs.gov/healthit/initiatives/

[13] Butz A, Kruger A (2006) User-centered development of a pervasive healthcare application. Proceedings of First International Conference on Pervasive Computing Technologies for Healthcare (IEEE), Nov.

[14] Weerasinghe D, Elmufti K, Rajarajan M, Rakocevic V (2006) XML security based access control for healthcare information in mobile environment. Proceedings of First International Conference on Pervasive Computing Technologies for Healthcare (IEEE), Nov.

[15] Ferreira A, Barreto L, Brandao P, Correia R, Sargento S, Antunes L (2006) A secure wireless architecture to access a virtual electronic patient record. Proceedings of First International Conference on Pervasive Computing Technologies for Healthcare (IEEE), Nov.

[16] Bui A, Aberle D, Kangarloo H (2007) TimeLine: visualizing integrated patient records. IEEE Trans Inf Technol Biomed. 11(4):462-73, July

[17] Katehakis D, Sfakianakis S, Kavlentakis G, Anthoulakis D, Tsiknakis M (2007) Delivering a lifelong integrated electronic health record based on a service oriented architecture. IEEE Trans Inf Technol Biomed. 11(6):639-650, Nov.

[18] Choi J, Yoo S, Park H, Chun J (2006) MobileMed: a PDA-based mobile clinical information system. IEEE Trans Inf Technol Biomed. 10(3):627-635, July

[19] Pohjonen H, Ross P, Blickman J, Kamman R (2007) Pervasive access to images and data—the use of computing grids and mobile/wireless devices across healthcare enterprises. IEEE Trans Inf Technol Biomed. 11(1):81-86, Jan

[20] Chu Y, Ganz A (2004) A mobile teletrauma system using 3G networks. IEEE Trans Inf Technol Biomed. 8(4):456-462, Dec.

[21] Toledo P, Jimenez S, Pozo F, Roca J, Alonso A, Hernandez C (2006) Telemedicine experience for chronic care in COPD. IEEE Trans Inf Technol Biomed. 10(3):567-573, July.

Chapter 3: Pervasive Computing and Healthcare

Abstract Pervasive computing technologies have seen significant advances in the last few years. This has resulted in design and development of sensors, wearable technologies, smart places and homes, and wireless and mobile networks. In this chapter, we first discuss current and emerging trends in pervasive computing and then present how pervasive computing can lead to pervasive healthcare. More specifically, examples of pervasive health monitoring, mobile telemedicine, intelligent emergency management service, health-aware mobile device, pervasive access to health information, pervasive life style management, and medical inventory management system are presented. We also identify various requirements of pervasive healthcare and present open issues and challenges to spur more research in this area.

3.1 Pervasive Computing

One of the most important quotes of all time in computing is from Mark Weiser who said, "The most profound technologies are those that disappear. They weave themselves into the fabric of everyday life until they are indistinguishable from it" [1]. This implies that technologies that get integrated so well in our life that they are no longer seen as separate entities or something different are likely to have the most impact or influence. This vision has become the foundation of almost all ubiquitous and pervasive computing work. Ubiquitous is something that is available anywhere anytime, while pervasive is something that is permeated in the environment. For this chapter, we consider both of these computing types together as shown in Figure 3.1. Here the access to computing and communications resources is ubiquitous, while many technologies such as sensors and devices have permeated in our environment. The four different implementations of the pervasive technologies are implanted, wearable, portable, and environmental. The level of indistinguishableness varies for each of these as implantable technologies may be completely invisible, wearable technologies may be somewhat visible, while portable technologies may be more visible. The environmental technologies, depending on the level of integration such as using a television for smart display, could also become indistinguishable.

U. Varshney, *Pervasive Healthcare Computing: EMR/EHR, Wireless and Health Monitoring*,   39
DOI: 10.1007/978-1-4419-0215-3_3,
© Springer Science + Business Media, LLC 2009

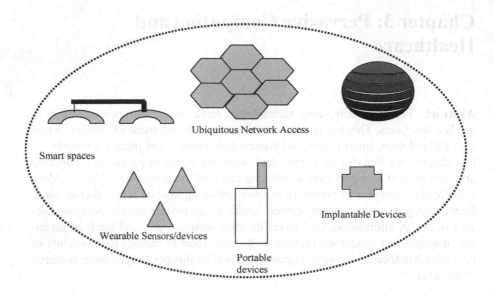

Fig. 3.1 Ubiquitous and Pervasive Computing

Taken together, **ubiquitous and pervasive computing** (UPC) is designed so

- A user could be as productive as possible in her tasks without being aware of or distracted by the complexity of its surroundings such as networks, devices, software, and databases. This means she can focus on her tasks and not on the finer details of the supporting environment.
- The intelligence in the system is to not allow user mobility and changes in the surroundings to make user become more aware of his environment. This means that mobility and other changes are handled so smoothly that he does not perceive these changes.
- The user does not have to know which network her information is being transmitted, which database or server is completing his/her transactions, how changes from one location to another affect bandwidth, processing, and security of the environment. This means that different pieces involved in processing are not visible to the user.

Some major challenges in ubiquitous and pervasive computing are (a) finding out user-Intent, (b) supporting context awareness, (c) providing energy management, and, (d) protecting user privacy and trust [2]. Also, the adaptation to changing computing and networking environment is a major challenge. Next, we elaborate on these challenges.

First, **user intent** is what the user is trying to accomplish by using pervasive and ubiquitous environment. Then the computing system can help the user by making suitable decisions on her behalf. In practice, deriving or finding out user intent is not an easy job, but as one of the goals of pervasive computing is to be minimally intrusive thus asking user what she wants to do is not the first option. So in many cases, the user intent must be derived based on user's past and current actions, location, identity and past history of use.

The user's context depends on physical location, physiological state, emotional state, personal history, and behavioral pattern. **Context-awareness** implies the awareness of user's state and surroundings by UPC system and modification of its behavior based on this context information. Also for achieving minimal intrusiveness, where the computing system does not appear to be intrusive on user activities or behavior, context-awareness would be very helpful for the system to assist the user without the user becoming aware of its environment.

Sophisticated capabilities in UPC environment require more battery power, but the reduced size of hand-held devices leads to restriction on battery size (and power). This clearly means that some form of **energy management** is required. This can be done in several different ways (Figure 3.2). The user devices can go to sleep cycle when not in use and periodically wakeup to do their processing work. During sleep, a device spends minimal energy, but is not able to receive any transmission thus requiring some other device to receive and store any information addressed for the device under sleep. A more frequent sleep will conserve more power. Also, the amount of memory that needs to be refreshed can be reduced to save power. Many of the UPC applications can switch to low power low quality (fidelity) mode to save power, especially if user intent or context is available. The devices could also receive some processing help from near-by smart spaces, thus saving energy even further. In practice, these techniques could be combined to produce greater energy savings. The battery charging could occur in many ways such as traditional electrical charging or in the future more thermal and/or solar charging.

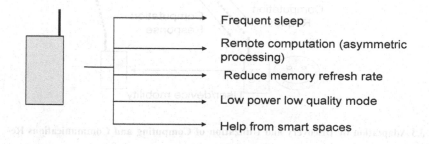

Frequent sleep

Remote computation (asymmetric processing)

Reduce memory refresh rate

Low power low quality mode

Help from smart spaces

Fig. 3.2 Several Ways for Energy Conservation and Management

Privacy is greatly complicated in pervasive and ubiquitous computing. Due to the monitoring of user actions, pervasive and ubiquitous system could become more aware of the user's behavior, intent, habits, actions, location, and movements. As the system knows so much about the user, there is a chance for potential misuse of this information ranging from spam to blackmail by hackers or others with access to this information. The potential loss of privacy may affect many users from using a pervasive and ubiquitous computing system or turning off their devices as soon as their tasks are completed.

Finally, **adaptation** to changing computing and networking environment is also very important in the UPC environment. With user mobility, the devices find themselves in environments that may have different set of computing and communication resources. The adaptation could involve both searching and utilizing the available computing resources (Figure 3.3) and making software and application changes in the new environment for adaptation (Figure 3.4). This assumes that computing resources are available and co-operative and mobile user is able to access them in his new location. The software and application changes are much more complex and involve moving the execution to another device or finding a co-operative device/server to assist in the processing.

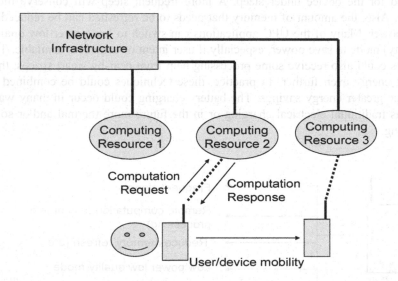

Fig. 3.3 Adaptation by Discovery and Utilization of Computing and Communications Resources

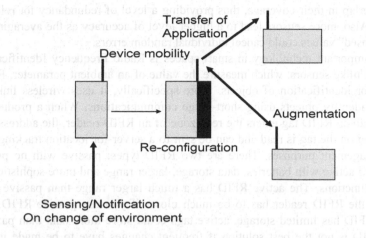

Fig. 3.4 Software and Application Changes for Adaptation

3.1.1 Smart Spaces

In simple terms, smart space is a space surrounded by technology that can sense and act, communicate, reason, and interact with people. This will allow people to be more productive and thus it is a preferred place to work and live. Thus in smart spaces, technologies are embedded in the environment and these interact with people. Why do we need smart spaces? As humans need to do more high-level and complex tasks, a large number of mundane and repetitive things can be done by technologies in smart spaces, and also smart spaces can help in doing more complex tasks. Currently several prototypes exist and could become available commercially in the near future in the form of smart products, smart displays, smart homes/houses, and smart cars.

Sensors are one of the most important technologies in smart spaces. These are small tiny devices with sensing, computation and wireless communications capabilities, but lack mobility. These used to be expensive, but manufacturing of small and low cost sensors has become technically and economically feasible now. Sensors measure ambient conditions in their surrounding environment and then transform these into signals. The signals can then be processed to determine the conditions of the "sensed" environment. The sensors could measure temperature, humidity, smoke, fire, leaks, gas, pressure, intruders among many other things. Although an individual sensor maybe sufficient for some applications, more and more distributed environments utilize sensor networks. Such networks may have hundreds or even thousands of sensors, where each sensor acts as a node and can communicate with its neighbors or a base station. In practice, multiple sensors could overlap in their coverage, thus providing a level of redundancy for reliable sensing. Also, more sensors lead to a higher level of accuracy as the averaging of more "sensed" values could cancel individual random errors.

Another important technology in smart spaces is Radio Frequency Identification (RFID). Unlike sensors, which measure the value of an ambient parameter, RFID is used for identification of objects. More specifically, it uses wireless links to uniquely identify objects using short-range communications. When a product or person with an RFID tag enters the read zone of an RFID reader, the address and data stored on the tag is read and can be sent to a server for location tracking and data management purposes. There are two RFID types: passive with no power source and active with batteries, data storage, larger range and more sophisticated security functions. The active RFID has a much larger range than passive one, meaning the RFID reader has to be much closer if you use passive RFID. Although RFID has limited storage, active tags could store more data than passive ones. RFID is not the best solution if frequent changes have to be made in the stored data. Also, although designed for very different purposes, RFID and sensors could work together for supporting different applications in smart spaces.

3.1.2 Smart House

The goal is to create assistive environments for older and/or disabled people such as homes, which can sense themselves and their residents. These can also enact mappings between the physical world and remote monitoring and intervention services. Although, there are several examples and implementations of smart houses now, we discuss Gator Tech Smart House (Figure 3.5) from University of Florida [3]. Some of the most fascinating features are smart blinds to control ambient light and to provide privacy; smart bed to monitor sleep patterns; smart closet to make clothing suggestions based on outdoor weather conditions; smart mirrors for messages and reminders for medications/tasks; smart bathroom with sensors for measurement of weight, height and temperature, and ECG; and SmartWave or a smart microwave that may refuse to heat-up specific items that you are not suppose to eat. There are also provisions for social-distant dining using immersive video, smart floor for fall detection, and cognitive assistant to guide occupants in tasks, such as cooking.

In the future, several features could be added to a smart house. The features may be what a person living in home or assisted living facilities would be benefitted the most. These could include personalized memory support applications, daily schedule management, medications reminders, context-aware assistant, smart first-aid, and, personalized entertainment services. As many of the residents of smart house are likely to have some cognitive decline or early dementia, it should have technologies to support in their daily tasks and activities.

One requirement of smart house is a very high level of reliability and the ability to work even under failures of some components. Only the catastrophic failures should be visible to the resident of Smart House. Even in those cases, it should cause no harm to the resident and inform the caregivers about the conditions of the house.

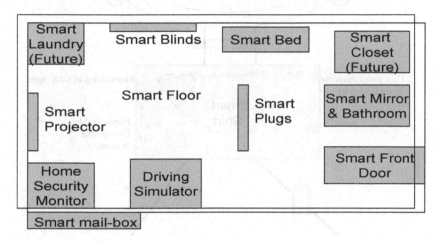

Fig. 3.5 Some Features of Gator Tech Smart House

3.1.3 Wearable Computing

Wearable computers are one part of the big vision of "Pervasive Computing", where people will have access to computing anywhere anytime. Wearable computing can support this by embedding computers in many daily-life components such as clothing, glasses, caps, headwear, shoes, and other wearable objects. In the future, a new generation of computers will become available that are designed as clothing items (Figure 3.6). Wearable computers will be designed to provide portability during operation, where people will access computing and communications functionality without being burdened by the weight and shape of computing devices. These devices will provide hands-free or virtually hands-free use, where people will be able to perform other tasks without being burdened by the need to hold or carry computers in their hands. The wearable computers will run continuously allowing the users to access them as and when necessary without a significant access delay. The wearable computers will attempt to sense the user's current context and will thus help him/her in performing the task effectively.

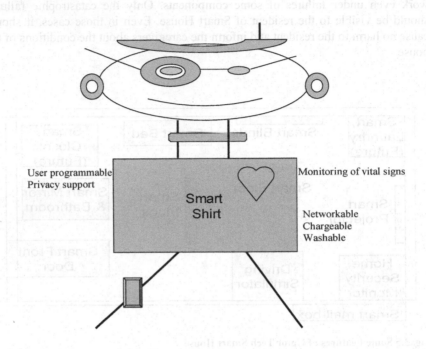

User programmable
Privacy support

Smart
Shirt

Monitoring of vital signs

Networkable
Chargeable
Washable

Fig. 3.6 Several Different Variation of Wearable Computers

The goal of wearable computing is an interface ideal for a continuously worn, intelligent assistant that augments memory, intellect, communication, and abilities [2]. The style of interface is the focus of wearable computing, as opposed to the manifestation in hardware as shown in media and other outlets [2]. The major challenges in wearable computers relate to [2]:

- power requirements,
- network resources,
- privacy concerns,
- innovative interfaces

A wearable computer can be a single worn device or a group of devices spread over the human body. This potential distribution of subsystems over the body could lead to very complicated power use and distribution. This distribution involves both how power is generated and dissipated by wearable computers. The wearable computers can have their batteries charged when a user is sleeping, eating, or driving. Alternatively, the human body could act as both a charger (source) for these devices as well as an end medium for heat absorption (sink).

The networking challenges in wearable computers are much more complex as both intra-body and inter-body communications may be supported in addition to communications to other networks. The intra-body communications can be supported by creating Body Area Networks (BANs) where individual subsystems on the human body can act as networking devices (such as routers). Depending on the frequency used, line of sight issues may have to be addressed. From a topology point of view, a wearable computing device in the center of human body can act as a switch or router and thus can minimize the power requirement for BANs. The inter-body communications to another similarly equipped human with wearable devices can be direct point-to-point or assisted by other humans (ad hoc networking) or could go through another wireless network covering both the source and destination humans. Both intra (on the same person) and inter (among different persons) body area networks are shown in Figure 3.7.

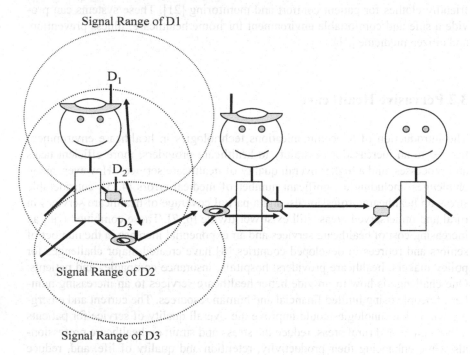

Fig. 3.7 Intra and Inter Body Area Networks (BANs)

Wearable computing generates a significant level of privacy concerns. Wearable computers could store a large amount of "intimate" information on users, thus creating privacy challenges. Hackers may find it very attractive to collect private information about everyone who passes by certain places in a city. In some cases, privacy may also be compromised by employers or co-workers. With wearable computers, a user should be informed what personal information is collected while passing by or accessing a certain network service. This would allow a user to make a benefit-loss tradeoff before allowing a location- or service-based function. In some cases, especially medical or emergency situations, privacy violations could be considered desirable and thus even be encouraged.

Interface refers to the numerous fields that address human and computer interaction. These fields include human-computer interfaces, human factors, ergonomics, industrial design, and fashion [2]. In the future, wearable computing can be implemented as a cross-section of multiple domains of engineering, design, and fashion. Also, the peripheral interfaces should be designed to make simple things simple and complex things possible [2].

Wearable computing can be applied for healthcare scenarios in many different locations and range of embedded sensors. Advances in many technologies such as low power design, new textiles, and flexible sensors would allow design of user-friendly clothes for patient comfort and monitoring [21]. These systems can provide a safe and comfortable environment for home healthcare, illness prevention, and citizen medicine [21].

3.2 Pervasive Healthcare

The introduction of telecommunications technologies in healthcare environment has led to an increased accessibility to healthcare providers, more efficient tasks and processes, and a higher overall quality of healthcare services. However, many challenges, including a significant number of medical errors [4, 5], considerable stress on healthcare professionals, and a partial coverage of healthcare services in rural and underserved areas, still exist worldwide [6, 7]. These combined with an increasing cost of healthcare services and an exponential increase in the number of seniors and retirees in developed countries [8] have created major challenges for policy makers, healthcare providers, hospitals, insurance companies and patients. One challenge is how to provide better healthcare services to an increasing number of people using limited financial and human resources. The current and emerging wireless technologies could improve the overall quality of service for patients in both cities and rural areas, reduce the stress and strain on healthcare professionals while enhancing their productivity, retention and quality of life, and, reduce the long-term cost of healthcare services. Many medical errors occur due to a lack of correct and complete information at the location and time it is needed, resulting in wrong diagnosis and drug interaction problems [4, 5]. The required medical information can be made available at any place any time using sophisticated devices and widely deployed wireless networks. Although, wireless technologies cannot eliminate all medical errors, but some of the informational-errors can certainly be eliminated by such access to medical information. The wireless technologies can be effectively utilized by matching infrastructure capabilities to health-care needs. These include the use of location tracking, intelligent devices, user interfaces, body sensors, and short-range wireless communications for health monitoring; the use of instant, flexible and universal wireless access to increase the accessibility of healthcare providers; and reliable communication among medical devices, patients, health-care professionals, and vehicles for effective emergency management. In the long-term, affordability, portability, and re-usability of wireless technologies for health monitoring and preventive care will also reduce the overall cost of healthcare services.

Next how wireless technologies have been introduced in healthcare is discussed. The use of wireless sensors in minimally invasive continuous health-monitoring systems is discussed in [9]. A maritime multi-lingual telemedicine system that uses satellite and ground-based networks for supporting audio and video-conferencing, and multimedia communications is presented in [10]. Several applications of wireless telemedicine systems including tele-cardiology, tele-radiology, and tele-psychology are presented in [11]. An implementation of pervasive computing technologies in an assisted-care facility (www.elite-care.com), where by using network sensors and databases, facility staff members are alerted when residents need immediate care, is presented in [12]. A wearable healthcare assistant has been designed to sense pulse waves, user's actions, and postures, and to capture contextual photos and continuous voice. A high-pressure (stressful) state is detected from the high pulse-rate by using the acquired context information [13]. The information is stored and retrieved on a website and requires modification for fitting on smaller handheld devices. It has been shown that the elderly are ready to begin using wireless technologies as long as these truly facilitate independent living [14]. An overview of general issues in m-health can be found in [15]. A description of "Personal Wellness Systems" and related technologies and usage scenarios is presented in [16].

The current use of wireless and mobile technologies in healthcare involves the use of pagers, hand-held devices, tablet PCs, and other computers to communicate with healthcare professionals and for access to patient information. This includes use of both wireless paging networks (combination of terrestrial and satellite networks) and wireless LANs. Increasingly, monitoring devices, including Smart Shirt, are becoming available for obtaining, recording and monitoring one or more vital signs such as blood pressure. Most of the current monitoring devices use wireline networks such as telephone networks. Many ongoing trials involve single medical applications and wireless access (Connected health at Harvard, Global Care Quest at UCLA medical school).

Currently, most hospitals/nursing homes lack wireless coverage (some even discourage it) and the others still dealing with reliability and coverage problems. There are many challenges, including real and "perceived" problems in wireless technologies, hand-held devices, and a level of privacy, which must be addressed before "pervasive healthcare" becomes a reality. So far, the introduction is quite preliminary without identifying healthcare requirements and challenges, limited utilization of the unique capabilities of wireless infrastructure, use of a single type of wireless network, thus restricting the access and coverage, and resulting in a very fragmented use.

In this section, a vision of pervasive healthcare is presented that includes applications and requirements of pervasive healthcare, wireless networking solutions and several important research problems. We define pervasive healthcare as "healthcare to anyone, anytime, and anywhere by removing locational, time and other restraints while increasing both the coverage and the quality of healthcare". This includes prevention, healthcare maintenance and checkups; short-term monitoring (home healthcare monitoring), long-term monitoring (nursing home), and personalized healthcare monitoring; and incidence detection and management, emergency intervention, and, transportation and treatment (Figure 3.8). The pervasive healthcare applications include pervasive health monitoring, intelligent emergency management system, pervasive healthcare data access, and ubiquitous mobile telemedicine. The wireless networking solutions include use of wireless LANs, ad hoc wireless networks, cellular/GSM/3G infrastructure-oriented networks and satellite-based systems.

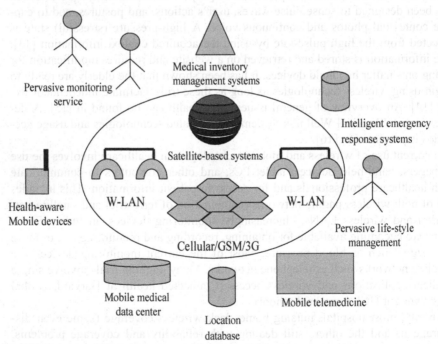

Fig. 3.8 Pervasive Healthcare and Several Applications

3.2.1 Mobile and Ubiquitous Telemedicine

Telemedicine, or the use of telecommunications technologies for medical diagnostics, treatment and patient care, has been in operation for several years, although on a limited scale [17]. Currently mobile devices such as PDAs with 802.11 wireless LAN access are being used to upload and download schedules for patients and doctors. In few places, doctors and nurses can access patient information on a PDA or hand-held devices and can also enter new information. People can be reminded of their appointments on their PDAs by displaying short text messages.

It is likely that mobile telemedicine services would be adopted on a wide scale. The reasons behind this optimism are (a) increasingly mobile savvy society with more than 3.5 billion handheld devices worldwide, (b) deployment of wireless-based solutions in developing countries where "wire-line" infrastructure is minimal or impractical, (c) portability and usability of mobile hand-held devices combined with an increasingly sophisticated workforce.

A possible scenario for the proposed architecture is as follows. A physician from an out-patient clinic prefers to go to a far away nursing home only if there are several patients for comprehensive evaluation. However, preliminary consultations with nursing home staff, patients, and other doctors could be done by using hand-held devices and access to multiple wireless networks, allowing her to be in a car, office, airport, traffic jam, or other places. The proposed architecture can be used to facilitate this scenario (Figure 3.9). Such a system will also enable an "information-aware" physician to download the necessary patient information before arriving at a nursing home.

The characteristics and requirements of mobile telemedicine include a range of short and long sessions for consultation, coordination of two or more locations, pervasive and ubiquitous access to patient data and information, and ability to transmit encrypted data, images, video and medical information. There may be other specific requirements based on the coverage and healthcare environment. The specific networking requirements include dependable and reliable network architectures, universal access to wireless networks, real-time support for information upload and download and discussions, support for significant quality of service, and continued access for sessions. The additional requirements include security and privacy, mobile devices that can work with minimal input requirements and have voice activation, and ways to support the installation and usage cost of mobile telemedicine systems. Maintainability and upgradability of telemedicine systems should also be addressed to allow long-term use.

There are also issues of the level of insurance payments for mobile telemedicine services rendered to patients, and potential mistakes, errors and liability issues. Although mobile telemedicine extends the range of healthcare coverage for patients, the quality of care and error reporting must also be addressed. More work is also needed in identifying the most suitable applications for mobile telemedicine, such as counseling and tele-psychiatry, and consultation. Additionally, there are challenges of cost, usability, market needs, reliability and patient safety.

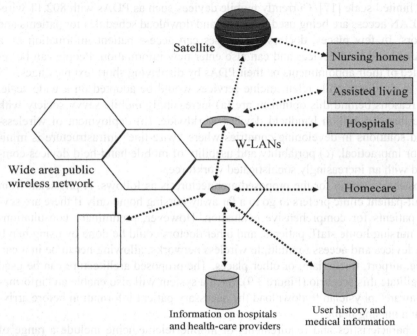

Fig. 3.9 An Architecture for Mobile Telemedicine

3.2.2 Pervasive Patient Monitoring Services

This application involves health monitoring of patients at anytime in any location. This could include homes, assisted living facilities, hospitals or nursing homes. Using his/her medical history and current conditions, one or more actions can be taken including sending an alert message to the nearest ambulance or a healthcare professional (Figure 3.10). These monitoring services could use location-tracking capabilities of wireless networks including satellites (for outdoor tracking) and cellular/wireless LANs (indoor). Also, some intelligence (context awareness) can be built in pervasive services to avoid "false-positive" alerts. The pervasive patient monitoring services could reduce the time between the occurrence of an emergency and the arrival of needed help.

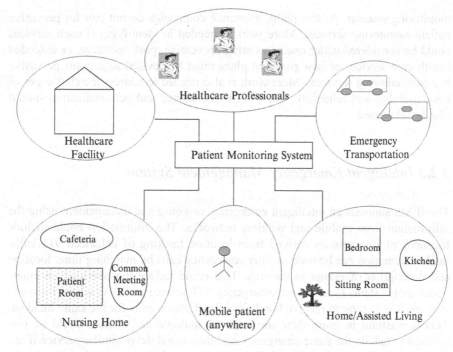

Fig. 3.10 Pervasive Health Monitoring Service

In general, the coverage of wireless networks is not comprehensive on every square meter of a facility. This could result in time and location-dependent dead-spots with unpredictable wireless coverage. Currently in a typical nursing home in USA, a patient is observed by a nurse or staff one to few times an hour. In between, if a patient goes to bathroom and start to have a serious medical condition such as heart attack, the required help may not come in time. By the time a nurse or staff comes again, it may be too late. Even if there was a wireless system to monitor, it may not have coverage in some areas where patient could go. To avoid this situation, use of multiple wireless networks could be considered.

The requirements of pervasive patient monitoring includes continuous monitoring for some patients and event-driven monitoring for others, the frequency of monitoring, number and types of vital signs that must be monitored and transmitted, and the size and frequency of messages to be transmitted. The specific networking requirements include universal access to wireless networks, location management, high-levels of wireless network reliability, network scalability with an increased number of users and frequency of monitoring, and support for prioritized transmission of vital signs of certain patients. The quality of service requirements are low delay and high probability of message delivery. The additional requirements include security and privacy, and ways to support the usage cost of mobile patient monitoring systems. At this point, insurance companies do not pay for pervasive patient monitoring services. More work is needed in identifying if such services could be considered under one of existing preventive, post-operative, or extended health care services or new payment plans must be devised to support pervasive health monitoring services. More work is also needed to address the challenges of cost, usability and reliability. The patient acceptance and personalization should also be addressed.

3.2.3 Intelligent Emergency Management System

The IEMS supports an intelligent emergency response and management using the information from mobile and wireless networks. The information could include locations of emergencies derived from location tracking of enhanced 911 calls. Such information can be used to filter emergency calls by matching time, location and description of events as patterns. This could reduce the overload on emergency call systems (such as the emergency 911 service in USA) where for some systems it is routine to receive hundreds of cell phone calls for the same incident. This is wasteful in more than one ways as multiple ambulances could be dispatched to handle the same emergency and thus could delay similar service if another incident takes place. The information from wireless networks can also be used to find the best routes by using the real-time traffic information and allowing inter-vehicular communication to update the traffic routing information (Figure 3.11). This could be combined with finding the closest hospital(s) with the needed care and also to check the availability of hospital space. If the information derived from the sensors on the bodies of people involved in emergencies can be processed, it may be possible to implement a prioritized healthcare delivery mechanism in routing of emergency vehicles. These intelligent additions would improve the overall efficiency of the emergency management system allowing it to maximize the number of emergency cases it can handle with a limited budget and people. The proposed changes can also result in saving many more lives while keeping the quality of service at high level for others.

The requirements of intelligent mobile emergency response system include support for inter-vehicle communications for incident management and for finding best-current-route for vehicles. How to maintain communications among vehicles moving at high-speeds and the short contact time for communications must be addressed. The quality of communications channel at high-speed and the amount of spectrum necessary for inter-vehicle communications must also be considered. It is also possible that communications among the emergency vehicles can be facilitated by emergency call system, but the network coverage and processing requirements could affect the scalability of such mediated communications. In some implementations, the system could communicate all the necessary information directly to emergency vehicles, thus not needing any communications among vehicles for emergency management. Other requirements include location-tracking of incidents, and automatic filtering of same incident-call by matching location, time and description of incidents. In terms of traffic, the sessions are likely to be short and unicast communication for callers and multicast for emergency vehicles must be supported. The specific networking requirements include location management for calling parties, incidents, and the emergency vehicles. Also, the wireless infrastructure must be dependable and support real-time communications among vehicles. The additional requirements are significant levels of intelligence in the emergency system and wireless networks, and scalability of the system as the number of users, incidents, calls, and vehicles are increased.

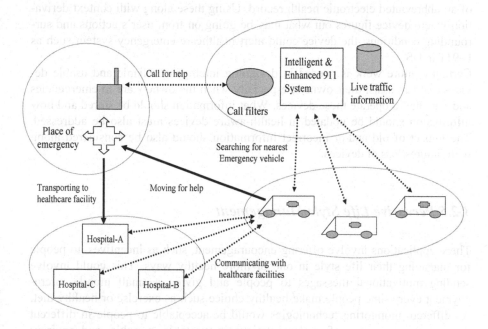

Fig. 3.11 Intelligent Emergency Management System

The Intelligent Emergency Management System should be very reliable and in any case should cause no harm to patients even under failures of one or more of its components. The human operators of this system should be able to override any of the automated decisions if they are convinced that the system is operating incorrectly or is relying on incorrect or incomplete information.

Many of the current traffic and health emergency management systems could evolve into such IEMS or similar systems. Many of the features of IEMS could also be implemented in the emerging Intelligent Transportation Systems (ITS).

3.2.4 Health Aware Mobile Devices

The capabilities of current and emerging mobile devices are continuously increasing with increased computing and communications power and increasing level of intelligence of hardware and software. Some of the devices have multi-network access, meaning these can access more than one type of wireless networks, such as wireless LANs and Bluetooth.

In future, mobile devices could become health-aware, where the devices could detect certain conditions by the touch of a user. This could include measurement of pulse-rate, blood pressure, level of alcohol. Also, some smaller medical devices can be integrated or added in the hand-held/wearable wireless device. The mobile devices can also store health history and all known medical conditions in the form of an abbreviated electronic health record. Using these along with context derivation where device figures out what may be going on from user's actions and surrounding conditions, the device could alert healthcare emergency system such as E-911 in US.

Certainly, more work is needed in designing intelligent, reliable and usable devices that can assist their owners, especially when the owners are in emergencies and not able to operate these devices. What information should be stored and how information should be updated in health-aware devices must also be addressed. The impact of old and/or incorrect information should also be considered along with failures/loss of devices.

3.2.5 Pervasive Life Style Management

These applications involve offering encouragement, such as incentives, to people for managing their life style in one or more healthy ways. This could involve sending motivational messages to people and giving a small mobile micro-payment every time people make healthy choice such as exercise or healthy diet. As different monitoring technologies would be acceptable to people in different demographics, a range of implementations in wearable, portable, and environmental forms could become possible. Some of these can automatically detect a range of exercises and/or activities, the people could still be asked to enter information to verify the actual activities of people in terms of when they are exercising or eating properly. The information can be entered by the user to mobile device in text, image or video form. Once verified, a suitable amount of mobile money is transferred to the device. This mobile money can then be used for paying wireless monthly charges, for donating to a charity of user's choice, or more importantly for paying healthcare expenses.

Such incentives can lead to healthier individuals and thus reducing the overall cost of healthcare services. Some companies are beginning to offer financial or other incentives for weight-loss/membership to health clubs. This may be more effective incentive than the proposed "fat tax" to recover the healthcare cost due to obesity, or increased penalty in the form of higher premiums for health insurance for people with weight problems.

3.2.6 Medical Inventory Management System

As stated before, many of the healthcare processes can be automated resulting in more efficiencies and possibly lower cost of healthcare services. Some of these can be facilitated by using specific features of wireless and mobile technologies. One example of how wireless location management techniques could be used in healthcare is shown in Figure 3.12, where medical inventories are managed using mobile devices. Although mobile inventory management systems are being deployed in other systems, the medical inventory in general is different. The particular characteristics are the nature of medications and supplies, need for authenticity, expiry dates, limited number of manufactures, a range of doses, presence of generic medications, and a certain quality needed for healthcare.

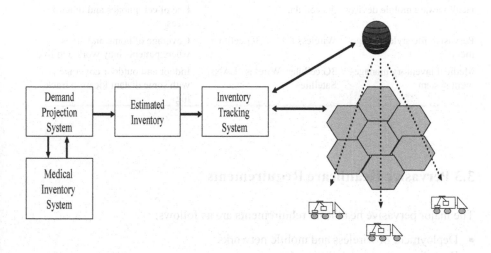

Fig. 3.12 Medical Inventory Management System

As the different supplies reach below a threshold as indicated by a wide-scale deployment of sensors, additional inventory is ordered and tracked using wireless networks. This system can be joined with demand projection system for "proactive" inventory management. Such an intelligent mobile inventory system is likely to reduce the cost of inventory while increasing the chances of finding a certain item when needed. To allow multiple suppliers to compete for medical supplies, mobile auction type trading can be performed, thus reducing the cost of supplies even further.

Using the characteristics and requirements of pervasive healthcare applications, it is possible to identify the suitable wireless networks for each application as shown in Table 3.1.

Table 3.1 Pervasive Healthcare Applications and Wireless Networks

Application	Suitable Wireless Networks	Comments
Mobile telemedicine	Satellites, 3G Cellular	The far away places and some bandwidth for communications
Pervasive patient monitoring services	Wireless LANs, Ad Hoc Networks, 3G cellular	Coverage of homes, hospitals, assisted living and mobile patients
Intelligent emergency management system	3G cellular, Satellites	E911 and distant coverage
Health aware mobile devices	3G cellular	Use of cell phones and other devices
Pervasive life style management	Wireless LANs, 3G cellular	Coverage of home and areas where patients may work and live
Medical inventory management system	3G cellular, Wireless LANs, Satellites	Indoor and outdoor coverage with some distant location tracking

3.3 Pervasive Healthcare Requirements

The major pervasive healthcare requirements are as follows:

- Deployment of wireless and mobile networks
- Pervasive access to healthcare data
- Highly secure communications
- High-level of privacy
- Highly reliable and usable infrastructure which is accessible, supports for prioritized communications, is always on by fault-tolerance, and has sufficient bandwidth

- A new business model on how much it will cost initially, different players and their roles, who will pay for it and how, and how would savings be used
- Insurance, liability, HIPAA, training and adoption

The diversity of wireless and mobile networks is a challenge in pervasive healthcare environment. The networks can cover from personal range (Bluetooth, RFID and Sensors) to short range (Wireless LANs and Ad Hoc networks) to wide range (Cellular-oriented wireless networks and Satellites). However, these networks use quite different technologies and protocols and are not able to inter-operate easily. There are some more challenges in pervasive healthcare. These include studying how pervasive healthcare can be implemented, offered and utilized. The training of healthcare professionals to use wireless and other IT systems would be required. More work is also needed in designing business models for pervasive healthcare and must address what cost items can be eliminated, what additional cost must be included, who will pay and incentives from federal government. While increasing the coverage of healthcare services, pervasive healthcare will also have to deal with new legal and regulatory issues and must consider insurance payments and cost aspects.

3.4 Open Issues and Challenges

There are many open issues and challenges in realizing the vision of pervasive healthcare. These include a lack of comprehensive coverage of wireless and mobile networks, reliability of wireless infrastructure, general limitations of handheld devices, medical usability of sensors and mobile devices, training of patients, interference with other medical devices, privacy and security, payment and many management issues in pervasive healthcare. It should be noted that use of pervasive healthcare applications would generate some controversy as privacy issues may become more challenging. The patients are likely to use pervasive healthcare systems if the information generated from them is accessed and used only by people they trust such as their healthcare professionals, care givers, and family members. More work is needed in addressing these challenges for pervasive healthcare. The technology issues related to pervasive healthcare includes networking support such as location tracking, routing, scalable architectures, dependability, quality of access, how to provide health monitoring in diverse environments (indoor, outdoor, hospitals, nursing homes, assisted living), continuous vs event-driven monitoring of patients, use of mobile devices for healthcare information storage, update, and transmission, sensing of vital signs and transmission using cellular networks and wireless LANs, formation of ad hoc wireless networks for enhanced monitoring of patients, managing healthcare emergency vehicles and routing and network support for mobile telemedicine. The design and development of comprehensive wireless health monitoring system should address challenges of reliability of wireless health monitoring. More work may also be needed in measuring any side-effects of having monitoring devices on patients for long-term monitoring. These may affect the adoption of pervasive healthcare.

The medical aspects are very important in realizing a wide-scale deployment of wireless in healthcare. The issues of how patient-care is delivered, how medical information can be represented, and requirements of diverse patients must be addressed. Many important issues are design of suitable healthcare applications, specific requirements of vital signs in healthcare environment, the diversity of patients and their specific requirements, representation of medical information in pervasive healthcare environment (multimedia, resolution, processing and storage requirements), role of medical protocols, improved delivery of healthcare services, and the usability of wireless-based solutions in healthcare. The requirements presented vary significantly from keeping track of the behavior of kids to how to avoid wandering and getting lost for dementia patients. It will be a major challenge to involve people with mental illness to use wireless infrastructure due to limited functional intelligence or very limited memory (such as those suffering from dementia). Many patients with paranoia may develop a suspicion towards wireless technologies, especially those once requiring a patient to wear a locator or other device. Some of the challenges could be overcome by providing training to patients on the usefulness and usability of the technologies for their care. As some patients may not become aware if their devices are malfunctioning or not working properly, such scenarios could be avoided by monitoring of devices by healthcare professionals and others. In future, the devices may have intelligence to check for any malfunction on their own.

The management of pervasive healthcare could bring a mini-revolution in terms of how wireless in the healthcare is implemented, offered and managed. There are many challenging and diverse management issues that must be addressed including the security and privacy in wireless healthcare, training of healthcare professionals for pervasive healthcare, managing the integration of wireless solutions, increasing coverage of healthcare services using wireless technologies, legal and regulatory issues, insurance payments and cost aspects, and the potential implications of HIPAA (Health Insurance Portability and Accountability Act of 1996). The usability and integration of wireless-based solutions in healthcare is another challenge. The devices must be designed to offer intuitive interfaces that can learn with and from individuals. It has been shown that many less-technical-savvy population segments are willing to learn and use mobile and wireless technologies for allowing them to live more independently. The training of healthcare professionals to effectively utilize mobile and wireless technologies would be a less complex issue as an increasing number of those are using hand-held and wireless devices. Another major issue is how to reduce the cost of delivering healthcare services to as many people by using wireless infrastructure. Other challenges in the large-scale introduction of wireless infrastructure in healthcare are legal and regulatory such as the issues of liability and law-suits in USA and possibility of insurance companies not paying or paying differently for treatment via mobile devices. Another major issue is privacy and possible misuse of patient medical information. In U.S., HIPAA, designed for protecting such information, has received some controversy and has been interpreted differently by major players, healthcare providers, insurance and attorneys. Therefore, work is needed in addressing privacy and related concerns over wireless and mobile networks where security is still seen as insufficient. It can be observed that ubiquitous and pervasive computing may add to the healthcare cost in the short-term, but will reduce the long-term cost especially when managing the chronic conditions. Before, many of the pervasive healthcare applications become reality, more work is needed in modifying financial and regulatory framework to support research, development, and deployment of technological solutions for pervasive healthcare.

Questions

1. How is pervasive computing different from ubiquitous computing? Why would one some one combine these two together?
2. What are some major challenges in UPC? Discuss your solutions and show why these could overcome major challenges?
3. Why being "not-intrusive" or "minimally intrusive" is a goal of UPC? What would happen if UPC is intrusive and user becomes aware of it?
4. What is a smart space? What roles can be played by sensors and RFID in smart space?
5. Suggest one application where sensors and RFID could work together.
6. Discuss two additional features, not covered in the text, in smart house.
7. In your opinion, what will be the biggest challenge in wearable computing and why?
8. What are some challenges in using wireless technologies in healthcare today?
9. Suggest and discuss one pervasive healthcare application of your choice that is not covered in the text.

References
[1] Weiser M (1991) The computer for the 21st century. Scientific American, 265(3): 94-104, September
[2] Starner T (2001) The challenges of wearable computing: Part 1. IEEE Micro 21(4): 44-52 and The challenges of wearable computing: Part 2. IEEE Micro 21(4): 54-67
[3] Helal S, Mann W, Zabadani H, King J, Kaddoura Y, Jensen E (2005) The Gator Tech smart house: a programmable pervasive space. IEEE Computer, 38(3): 64-74, March
[4] US Institute of Medicine Report "To Err Is Human: Building a Safer Health System" (http://www.nap.edu/books/0309068371/html/)
[5] JAMA Abstract "Estimating Hospital Deaths Due to Medical Errors," July 25, 2001 (vol. 286, issue 4) (http://jama.ama-assn.org/issues/v286n4/rfull/joc02235.html#abstract)
[6] Singh M (2002) Treating health care. IEEE Internet Computing, 6(4): 4-5, July-August

[7] Parsloe C (2003) Worlds apart? healthcare technologies for lifelong disease management. IEEE Engineering in Medicine and Biology Magazine, 22(1): 53-56, January-February

[8] US Administration on Aging Report on Demographic Changes, available at http://www.aoa.dhhs.gov/aoa/stats/aging21/demography.html

[9] Boric-Lubecke O, Lubecke V (2002) Wireless house calls: using communications technology for health care and monitoring. IEEE Microwave Magazine, 3(3): 43-48, Sept

[10] Anogianakis G, Maglavera S, Pomportsis A (1998) Relief for maritime medical emergencies through telematics. IEEE Transactions on IT in Biomedicine, 2(4): 254-260, Dec.

[11] Pattichis C, Kyriacou E, Voskarides S, Pattichis M, Istepanian R, Schizas C (2002) Wireless telemedicine systems: an overview. IEEE Antennas and Propagation Magazine, 44(2): 143-153, April

[12] Stanford V (2002) Using pervasive computing to deliver elder care. IEEE Pervasive Computing Magazine, 1(1): 10-13, Jan-March

[13] Suzuki T, Doi M (2001) LifeMinder: an evidence-based wearable healthcare assistant. In Proc. ACM Conference on Human Factors in Computing Systems, 127-128, March-April

[14] Mikkonen M, Vayrynen S, Ikonen V, Heikkila M (2002) User and concept studies as tools in developing mobile communication services for the elderly. Springer-Verlag's Personal and Ubiquitous Computing, 6: 113-124

[15] Guest Editorial (2004) M-Health: beyond seamless mobility and global wireless healthcare connectivity. IEEE Transactions on IT in Biomedicine, 8(4): 405-413, Dec.

[16] Dishman E (2004) Inventing wellness systems for aging in place. IEEE Computer, 37(5): 34-41, May

[17] Ogawa M, Togawa T (2003) The concept of home health monitoring. In Proc. of 5th International Workshop on Enterprise Networking and Computing in Healthcare Industry (Healthcom-2003)

[18] Varshney U (2003) Pervasive healthcare, IEEE Computer, 36(12): 138-140, Dec.

[19] Varshney U (2005) Pervasive healthcare: applications, challenges and wireless solutions. Communications of the AIS, 16(3), July

[20] Varshney U (2006) Using wireless technologies in healthcare. Int. Journal on Mobile Communications, 4(3): 354-368

[21] Axisa F, Schmitt P, Gehin C, Delhomme G, McAdams E, Dittmar A (2005) Flexible technologies and smart clothing for citizen medicine, home healthcare, and disease prevention. IEEE Transactions on IT in Biomedicine, 9(3): 325-336, Sept.

Chapter 4: Wireless and Mobile Technologies

Abstract In this chapter, wireless technologies and networks are presented. These include cellular networks, wireless LANs, satellites, sensors, RFID, Bluetooth, ZigBee and Fixed wireless networks. More specifically, the characteristics of different wireless networks are presented, and how wireless networks can be used in health monitoring is shown. It is also shown how their individual characteristics would affect their suitability for wireless health monitoring.

For better readability, the acronyms used in this chapter are shown in Table 4.1.

Table 4.1 The List of Acronyms Used

Acronym	Expanded Name
1G, 2G, 3G, 4G	First, Second, Third and Fourth Generation
AP	Access Point
BS	Base Station
DSSS	Direct Sequence Spread Spectrum
EDGE	Enhanced Data rate for GSM Evolution
FHSS	Frequency Hopping Spread Spectrum
GPRS	General Packet Radio Service
GSM	Group System for Mobile communications
HLR	Home Location Register
IEEE	Institute of Electrical and Electronics Engineers
IMT	International Mobile Telephony
ISM	Industrial, Scientific and Medical Band
ITU	International Telecommunications Union
LAN	Local Area Network
MSC	Mobile Switching Center
OFDM	Orthogonal Frequency Division Multiplexing
PSTN	Public Switched Telephone Network
RFID	Radio Frequency Identification
TDMA	Time Division Multiple Access
TDOA	Time Difference of Arrival
VLR	Visitor Location Register

U. Varshney, *Pervasive Healthcare Computing: EMR/EHR, Wireless and Health Monitoring,*
DOI: 10.1007/978-1-4419-0215-3_4,
© Springer Science + Business Media, LLC 2009

4.1 Introduction

The advances in wireless technologies have led to the design, development and deployment of several different mobile and wireless networks [1]. The number of "revenue generating" wireless handheld devices have already exceeded 3 billion worldwide [2]. In the next few years, wireless and mobile technologies will become location-aware, user preference-oriented and context-aware, and will be fully integrated in clothing, appliances, vehicles, grocery stores, individual items, books, and glasses among many diverse items. With these, wireless networks will play a major role in wireless health monitoring and pervasive healthcare [3, 4, 5]. What makes it challenging is the diversity of the current and emerging wireless and mobile networks [5, 6]. Some of these are personal area networks, such as Bluetooth and ZigBee, some are even shorter range such as RFID, some are local area networks such as wireless LANs, and some wide area networks such as cellular/3G and satellites. These networks also differ in the frequency they use, protocols they use for bandwidth, devices for access, and have peculiar characteristics. In general, the needed power for transmission is the square of the used frequency and also at least the square of the distance. With lots of buildings and obstacles, the power requirement could go up to the third or fourth power of the distance. Wireless networks also face a variety of problems inherent in wireless links, such as attenuation, slow fading, fast fading and multi-path interference (Figure 4.1). These problems affect the quality of transmission and reception and also limit the amount of information which can be transmitted over wireless links.

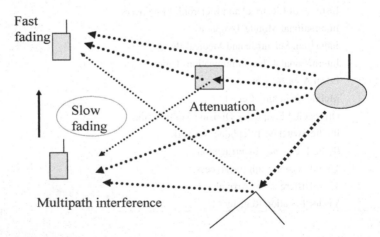

Fig. 4.1 Various Problems in Wireless Communications

Wireless networks can be designed for infrastructure or ad hoc configuration. The infrastructure configuration involves fixed network architecture and the user mobility is supported by handoff among base stations. In ad hoc network, the network configuration is not fixed and user communications is supported by co-operation of other devices, which act as routers. Both of these configurations are shown in Figure 4.2.

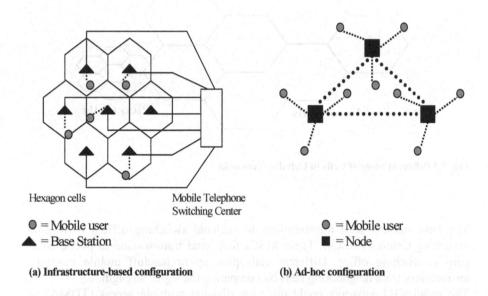

Hexagon cells   Mobile Telephone
                            Switching Center

◐ = Mobile user   ◐ = Mobile user
▲ = Base Station   ■ = Node

(a) Infrastructure-based configuration   **(b) Ad-hoc configuration**

Fig. 4.2 Infrastructure and Ad Hoc Configurations for Wireless Networks

4.2 The Commercial Cellular/3G Networks

The commercial cellular networks exist in several different generations, primarily in second (2G) and third generation (3G) now. They use radio signals between 1800-2200 MHz spectrum, with bands of frequencies allocated worldwide for specific implementations of local/global standards. The basic architecture of these commercial networks is cellular, where radio antennas are located throughout a service area with the range of each antenna, known as base station, constituting a "cell". The size of cells is influenced by the number of users and the need to reuse the limited frequency spectrum. Each cell can use a certain part of the spectrum and thus more cells (or smaller cells) are desirable to increase the reuse of spectrum. Generally cells are started as macro/micro cells covering several blocks or a mile of radius, but as the number of users is increased, the cells are made smaller (by adjusting the power of base station) to support more users in a given area (shown in Figure 4.3).

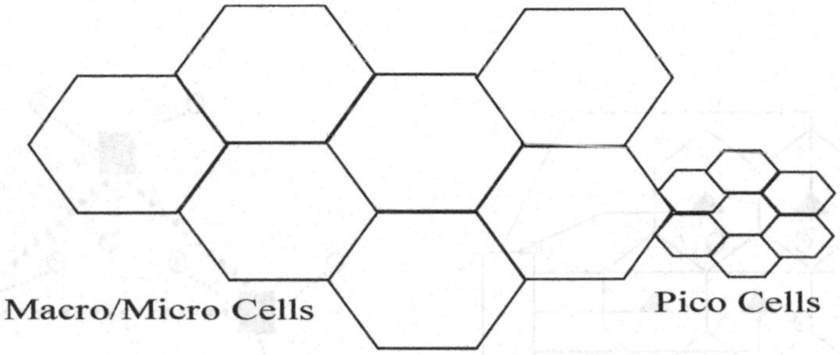

Macro/Micro Cells   Pico Cells

Fig. 4.3 Different Sizes of Cells in Cellular Networks

The base stations send transmissions to regional switching offices or Mobile Switching Centers (MSCs). These MSCs then send transmission to phone company's switching office. Different cells pick up or handoff mobile transmitter/receivers from neighboring cells by comparing the signal strength.

The cellular/3G networks could use time division multiple access (TDMA) or code division multiple access (CDMA) as their network access technique. There are several variations of these techniques resulting in a large number of different implementation worldwide, some of which support high-speed data transmission.

4.2.1 Existing Implementations

Worldwide cellular networks include 1G or analog cellular (829-894 MHz), digital cellular (same frequencies as analog cellular but each channel shared by three users), two versions of 2G networks based on time (1850-1990 MHz) or code division multiple access (1800-2000 MHz). Europe has been able to deploy and use a common standard, Global System for Mobile Communications (GSM), a variation of TDMA for its wide area cellular service (1710-1880 MHz). Time Division Multiple Access (TDMA) allocates a time slot to a mobile user and has been used in digital cellular, TDMA-based digital networks, and GSM networks. Code Division Multiple Access (CDMA) allocates a code sequence to a mobile user. Over time, several versions of CDMA have become standards. To support the need for higher bandwidth, 3G is using wideband CDMA and other CDMA variations, such as CDMAOne or CDMA2000. These are designed to provide fairly high-speed wireless communications to support multimedia, data, and video in addition to traditional voice traffic.

ITU's International Mobile Telecommunications for the year 2000 (IMT-2000) initiative defined third-generation capabilities to include 144 kbps to users in vehicles over large areas, 384 kbps to pedestrians over small areas, and 2.048 Mbps for office use with mostly fixed users or slowly moving users. 3G also have the flexibility to support introduction of new services and technologies to allow for 4G. Currently, the 4G networks are under development and several access schemes are being tested.

So it can be seen here that one factor that has been an obstacle in widespread deployment of wireless technologies is the existence of multiple "un-interoperable" standards and products. Although users in one network can communicate with users in another network using backbone such as PSTN, multiple cellular and wireless standards in US alone complicate the wireless usage. Multiple standards making interoperability much more difficult and limits the roaming between networks as cell phones using one of the access technologies (such as TDMA) cannot access other networks with different access technologies. The presence of multiple standards also slows down the development of new features and increases the chance that a user cannot access the services of a wireless network that is incompatible with its phone. The ways to improve are development and adoption of universal standard, use of multi-band and multi-adapter devices and design of a universal mobile device capable of translating the access protocol code. There has been progress in each of these three directions but have not been used widely.

4.2.2 Some Interesting Services

In addition to using a channel or code for making voice call, there are several other services that are offered and are of some interest to wireless health monitoring community. These include:

1. Short Messaging Service that allows GSM users to transmit short messages of up to 160 characters. These messages are stored & delivered in few seconds to minutes (not real-time delivery). SMS supports international roaming, thus heavily used for e-mail, voice mail and paging purposes and is the most popular GSM service. Several improvements are in progress such as increased message length, multiple messages per user at the same time and creation of distribution lists. SMS could be used in wireless health monitoring as reminders, messages, or in some cases as compressed information on patient's condition.

2. General Packet Radio Service (GPRS) is a packet data service by GSM and can support up to 160 Kbps. It also supports a mobile user's access to many different packet networks. GPRS supports Quality of Service and dynamic IP address allocation. It can be used in lots of countries due to the GSM availability in most continents. This is currently being offered in many US cities as some major carriers are introducing GSM/GPRS for high-speed data transmission.

3. Enhanced Data rate for GSM Evolution (EDGE) is considered a 2.5G technology due to its usage as a transition technology to the emerging 3rd generation wireless systems. EDGE can support up to 384 Kbps (using 600 KHz bandwidth) by using the link quality control, which adapts the error control technique to the current channel quality.

3G specifications offer the flexibility needed by both the existing operators to evolve their first and second-generation networks towards 3G services and the satellite/terrestrial providers in designing new 3G systems. The radio specifications allow five different choices, carefully designed to help existing first and second-generation wireless systems to interwork with or evolve into 3G systems. However, the worldwide migration to 3G took longer due to the operators' perception of market needs, lack of incentives to carriers and operators, investment made in the existing first and second generation wireless systems, and monopoly wireless carriers in many countries.

4.2.3 The Emerging 4G Networks

To support roaming across heterogeneous wireless networks (and not just across one type of wireless networks), very high bit rates for multimedia services, and packet-switched wireless communications, there is growing interest in the design and development of 4G wireless networks. The 4G wireless networks will allow users to move from one type of wireless network to another. For example, when the user is at home he/she can use the device as cordless phone to access PSTN. When in the car, he connects to a cellular network. While in an area not covered by such service, he can switch to a satellite-based network. After reaching to the office, he can switch to a high bandwidth Wireless LAN. The factors that distinguish the 4G networks are: the roaming across cellular, wireless LANs, Wireless WANs, satellites and other networks; IP interoperability; and higher bit rates in the range of 50 Mbps or more. The 4G networks are beginning to see some interests among researchers and vendors. While 3G networks are currently being deployed, 4G networks are expected in 2010 and beyond. Hopefully, this time frame gives everyone ample time to sort out differences and technical challenges. A comparison of the four generations is shown in Table 4.2.

Table 4.2. Different generations of commercial cellular networks

The Genera-tion	Key Features and Access	Access Protocols
1G (first generation)	Analog, primarily voice communications and some support for low rate data Supports access to and roaming across single type of analog wireless networks	Frequency Division Multiple Access (FDMA), where each user is assigned a channel for the duration of the call
2G and 2.5G (second generation)	Digital, secure, voice and data Supports access to and roaming across single type of digital wireless network Supports access to 1G networks	Time division Multiple Access (TDMA), where a user time-shares a channel or Code Division Multiple Access (CDMA), where a user is assigned a code for the duration of the call
3G (third generation)	Multimedia Supports global roaming across a single type of wireless network (e.g. cellular), 384 Kbps to several Mbps Supports access to 2G networks	TDMA and several variations of CDMA including Wideband CDMA are in use
4G (fourth generation)	Supports global roaming across multiple high bandwidth wireless networks, 50 Mbps or even higher, IP interoperability for seamless access to mobile Internet Access to 3G, and 2G networks	Several access techniques under development and testing for high bandwidth support

In 4G networks, the access to multiple wireless networks could also be facilitated by the use of an overlay network or by having intelligence in the networks. This would avoid having multiple interfaces or adapters in user devices. A possible scenario is shown in Figure 4.4, where common access points are used to allow a wireless device to access several different wireless networks. Such network architecture will allow a very high level of reliability for wireless health monitoring. This can overcome time and location-dependent access problems and/or failures in wireless networks.

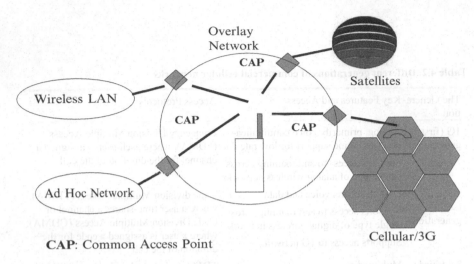

CAP: Common Access Point

Fig. 4.4 Accessing Multiple Wireless Networks

4.2.5 Location Management

The commercial cellular/3G networks use location management at two different levels. The higher level of location management is done to find the cell, where a certain phone is currently located. This is done for setting up a connection to that phone (shown in Figure 4.5). This involves user moving to a new area, registering with the database of that area (VLR), this VLR informing the home database of the user (HLR), and the HLR informing the database of user's previous location. The connection-setup involves the calling user entering the phone number of called user, MSC figuring out and contacting the called user's database (HLR), which in turn talks to the current database of the called user (VLR), then HLR sending information back to calling MSC. Then the connection between calling and called MSC is completed.

The lower level of location management, as required by FCC for enhanced 911 (E911) but not supported by all carriers in all locations yet, is to find more precise location of a phone (user) in cases of emergency [8]. This is shown in Figure 4.6. The E911 location tracking could be implemented using one of several techniques including time difference of arrival (TDOA) based on time differences (thus distance) in signals from a phone to reach to at least three neighboring base stations. Assisted GPS is another technology that is being used in cellular networks detecting caller's location and sending emergency help.

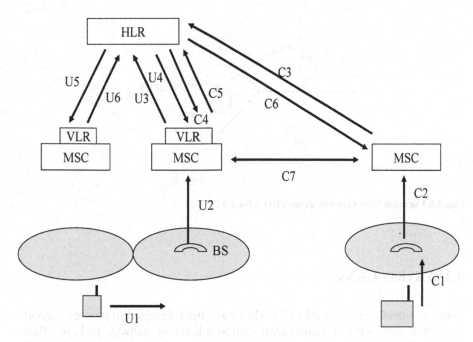

HLR: Home Location Register, VLR: Visitor Location Register

Update Process
U1: User moving to new area
U2: User registering with VLR
U3: VLR sending request to HLR
U4: HLR sending ACK to VLR
U5: HLR informing the old VLR
U6: Old VLR sending acknowledgement to HLR

Call Setup Process
C1: User making a call
C2: BS forwards the request to MSC
C3: MSC contacts HLR of the called user
C4: HLR contacts VLR of the called user
C5: VLR responds to HLR
C6: HLR sends calling VLR location information
C7: Calling and called MSCs finish the call set up

Fig. 4.5 Location Management for Completing Calls

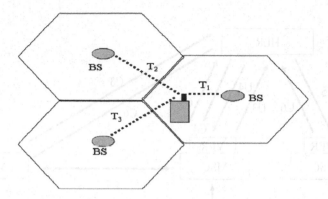

Fig. 4.6 Location Management using TDOA for E911

4.3 Wireless LANs

Wireless Local Area Networks (WLANs) have been designed to provide support for mobile computing in a small area, such as a building, hallway, park, or office complex. These can be designed for both infrastructure (central access point covering users in an area) and ad-hoc (peer-to-peer communications without an access point) configurations. The wireless LANs can provide wireless connectivity to hosts (computer, machinery, or systems) that require rapid deployment in a local area environment. These hosts can be stationary, portable, or mobile and may be hand-held or mounted on a moving vehicle. The primary uses of WLANs have been LAN extension, nomadic access in hot spots and broadband access to the Internet.

4.3.1 ISM Bands and Standards

Unlike cellular networks where a frequency or channel is allocated, users in WLANs have to share frequencies. One of the biggest issues for WLANs has been the spectrum availability. There are ISM (Industrial Scientific and Medical) bands in 902-928 MHz (U.S.), 2400-2483.5 MHz (Worldwide), and 5725-5850 MHz (U.S.). There are other ISM bands in 12 and 60 GHz also. The use of ISM bands, primarily the 2400-2483.5 MHz band, has always been the first choice. This has led to the original 802.11, 802.11b and now 802.11g standards for wireless LANs. The original 802.11 standard also included infrared as one of the transmission method. As the ISM bands were designated for unlicensed commercial use and are widely used by ambulances, police cars, taxicabs, and Citizen Band (CB) radios, there have been significant and varying levels of interference in some places from other users and also from many household and office devices operating in ISM bands, especially in 2.4 GHz. Even within a household, considerable interference could exist due to cordless phones, microwave ovens, and remote control toys. Security problems in general are due to the increased vulnerability due to open-air transmission, difficulty in encryption with smaller devices with somewhat limited abilities and weaknesses in many wireless standards (such as IEEE 802.11).

In addition to an increasing interference in this band, the demand for higher bit rates has also led to the consideration of other wider ISM bands for wireless LANs. IEEE 802.11a is a standard in the 5 GHz band, but as all other versions of 802.11 in use are in 2.4 GHz, the backward compatibility has been an issue. The use of dual-band LAN cards is possible but has not become widespread. In addition to the amount of bandwidth available in a spectrum and the level of interference present, the choice of spectrum also affects power requirement and the range. In general, power required is at least the square of the frequency and also square of the range (coverage). So, for example, 5 GHz based wireless LANs would require significantly more power, or at least 4 times higher, than 2.4 GHz wireless LANs for the same range (coverage area), or will lead to much smaller range for the same power. With many physical layer enhancements including coding of bits and better antenna design, energy efficient LAN protocols can reduce, but not eliminate, non-linear growth in power requirements at higher frequencies. In addition to multiple standards of IEEE 802.11, there are other standards for wireless LANs such as European HIPERLAN. Although designed for similar environment, these standards differ in frequency, bit rates, power requirements, and coverage. For example, 802.11, 802.11b and 802.11g use 2.4 GHz, while HIPERLAN is for 5.15-5.30 GHz. 802.11 WLAN supports 1 and 2 Mbps, while 802.11b supports 5 and 11 Mbps, and 802.11a (5 GHz) and 802.11g (2.4 GHz) go up to 54 Mbps. The main attraction is the flexibility and mobility that is supported by a wireless LAN and the bandwidth considerations have been secondary.

4.3.2 Mobility of Users

Wireless LANs do support mobility of user, where a user could move from one access point (AP) to another access point (Figure 4.7). This requires "disassociation" from the previous AP and "re-association" with the new AP. The user could communicate with the next AP to perform re-association and with the previous AP to perform disassociation. There may be a delay before this can be performed and in some cases, the user could reach to an area not covered by any of the access points of the wireless LAN. Several protocol solutions have been proposed to reduce the length of time during which user connectivity is interrupted after a move.

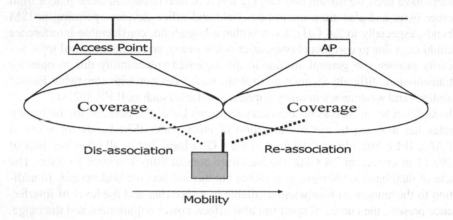

AP: Access Point

Fig. 4.7 User Mobility in Wireless LAN

4.3.3 Primary use of 802.11

IEEE 802.11 is used primarily for data applications as it was not designed to support real time traffic such as voice and video due to delay and bandwidth considerations. In future, the situation could change as attempts are being made to support packetized voice with echo cancellers and to increase the bit rate for high-speed real-time traffic. Although wireless LANs were originally designed as LAN extension and nomadic access for mobile users, now they are being deployed in hot-spots and switching among WLANs and cellular networks is started. Wireless LANs could become a vehicle for broadband access to the Internet.

4.3.4 Multiple Versions of 802.11

Although original 802.11 allowed three different ways to transmit data over the wireless channel such as frequency hopping spread spectrum (FHSS), Direct sequence spread spectrum (DSSS) and infrared, other versions have focused on a single method of transmission. For example, 802.11b only allows DSSS, while 802.11a uses orthogonal frequency division multiplexing (OFDM), a multi-carrier technique, where up to 52 carriers are used to transmit data from a single source to achieve 54 Mbps channel bit rate. A comparison of several different wireless LANs is shown in Table 4.3 [4]. As 802.11a uses different spectrum (wider and less crowded), one problem is that it is not "inherently" backward compatible to 802.11b (although use of dual-band adapters allowing access to both 80211.a and 802.11b/802.11g could address this problem). 802.11a signals travel less distance with same power, thus requiring more access points to cover the same hot-spot area (thus significantly affecting the economic survivability of carriers offering access in hot-spots). IEEE 802.11g is backward compatible with 802.11b as it uses the same 2.4 GHz band and provides the higher bit rates of 802.11a. Dual band adapters combining 802.11a, b, and g are available.

Table 4.3 The Multiple Versions of 802.11 for Communications

The version → Characteristics	802.11	802.11b	802.11a	802.11g
Spectrum used	2.4 GHz (ISM)	2.4 GHz (ISM)	5 GHz (ISM)	2.4 GHz (ISM)
Backward compatible with	None	802.11	None	802.11 and 802.11b
Protocol for Transmission	Frequency Hopping or Direct Sequence Spread Spectrum (FHSS or DSSS)	Direct Sequence Spread Spectrum (DSSS) only	Orthogonal Frequency Division Multiplexing (OFDM)	Orthogonal Frequency Division Multiplexing (OFDM)
Max. physical rate possible	2 Mbps	11 Mbps	54 Mbps	54 Mbps
Major disadvantage	Limited bit rate	Bit rate not enough for emerging applications	Smallest range of all 802.11 standards	Limited number of co-located wireless LANs
Major advantage(s)	Higher range	Widely deployed High range	Higher bit rate in a less crowded spectrum	Higher bit rate in 2.4 GHz Higher range than 802.11a
The current status	Being phased out	Widely Used	Limited use	Widely used

4.3.5 The future standards

The next version of wireless LANs is expected to be IEEE 802.11n. The maximum bit rate is expected to be as high as 540 Mbps and up to 50 meters, however more realistically it is likely to be between 100 and 200 Mbps. The higher bit rates will be achieved by using MIMO (Multiple-inputs and multiple-outputs) antennas along with specialized coding schemes. This allows multiple streams of data to be transmitted and received among network devices. It may operate in 2.4 and/or 5 GHz. There are many challenges including (a) backward compatibility with 802.11a, b, or g and (b) delays in completed standard (now expected in late 2009). Also, the primary impact on healthcare environment is likely to be the ability to transfer at higher bit-rate, support for more patients, and possibly improved security.

4.3.6 Suitability for Monitoring

Wireless LANs have several characteristics that make them suitable for wireless health monitoring in homes, assisted living facilities or nursing homes. First, wireless LANs provide coverage to support several rooms or even a floor. Second, wireless LANs are easy to install and have also become cheaper due to mass production of access points. Once installed, a wireless LAN does not involve any usage charges for users within the LAN, but may require some charges for accessing the Internet. Wireless LANs can support prioritized transmission of vital signs and related information, although these do not support real-time service. These characteristics have led to some interest in installing and using wireless LANs for health monitoring. In some cases, wireless LAN could be used just as the front-end of monitoring infrastructure, which then also utilizes another wireless network, such as the commercial cellular/3G network, as the back-end to connect to one or more healthcare professionals.

4.4 Satellites

Satellites use microwave signals, but as these signals are going in the air, thus not affecting any terrestrial objects, the frequency used can be higher. Many satellites today are using 40-60 GHz frequencies. Satellites can be thought of as a "microwave relay" station in the sky, where ground signal is received, then its frequency is moved to another band, usually a lower frequency band to conserve the power transmitted and then broadcasted towards the earth. There are many different types of satellites: geo-synchronous earth orbit (GEO at 22,300 miles above earth) satellites that remain stationary with respect to earth. Then low earth orbit (LEO at 300-1000 miles above earth) satellites with usually two-three hour rotational time. Then medium earth orbit (MEO) satellites exist between LEOs and GEOs and take few hours as their rotational time (Figure 4.8). As there are only 180 GEO satellites possible, the orbit is always limited. Besides orbit (height and rotational time), which also decides distance and delay to ground-based receivers, other major issues in satellite communications are power requirements, spectrum to be used, number of satellites, number of users, type of service (data, voice, paging) and size of receiver.

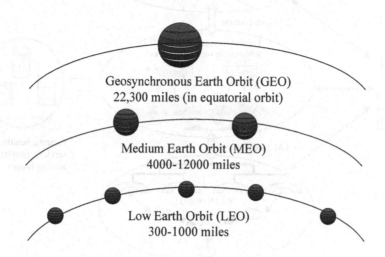

Fig. 4.8 Three Major Types of Satellites

There are many satellite-based systems that are in use including Global Position-ing Systems (GPS), Globalstar, Inmarsat (www.inmarsat.com), and Intelsat (www.intelsat.com). Many major failures include Motorola's IRIDIUM. Satellites could be used for mobile and wireless communications, however the recent fail-ures of many satellite-based projects have led to significant loss of interest in such services.

Geosynchronous satellites are in wide use providing broadcasting services, long distance and international phone services (to stationary users), paging services (to mobile/stationary users), and data networking services. However, with advances in antenna design, signal reception, and other related technologies, it is becoming possible to provide mobile services using satellites. Satellites can be used alone or in conjunction with other wireless networks in providing location management (Figure 4.9).

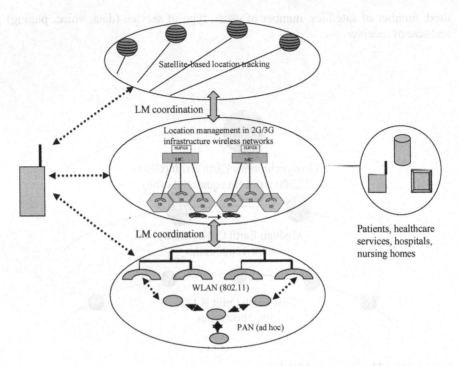

Fig. 4.9 Using Satellites with Other Networks to Provide Location Management

4.4.1 Satellites for Monitoring

The satellites can be used in wireless health monitoring. The advantages are broad coverage and the ability to broadcast the same information to multiple places. The disadvantages are limited uplink bandwidth between patients and satellites, primarily outdoor coverage, and high cost of access including bulky satellite devices. The satellites are also affected by weather conditions, including snow and rain. Wireless patient monitoring systems can be designed by taking into account these advantages and limitations of satellites. These could utilize satellites as the primary or secondary wireless network when other networks are not reachable. In many countries where neither wireline nor cellular wireless networks exist widely, satellites may be an option for wireless health monitoring. In some cases, access to a satellite is available only with some restrictions such as the need to have a clear view of southern skies for people living in the northern hemisphere. Also, the use of satellite antenna whether built-in a smart shirt or other monitoring device could make it more obvious to other people due to size and shape.

4.5 Sensors

Sensors are small devices with sensing, computation and wireless communications capabilities. The individual sensors are also known as sensor nodes, especially when used in a sensor-network. The sensors are usually kept in a place or location and thus are not mobile during their operation. With advances in technologies and demand for sensors in a range of application domains, manufacturing of small and low cost sensors has become technically and economically feasible now. The sensors measure ambient conditions in their surrounding environment and then transform these into signals, which can be processed to determine the conditions of the "sensed" environment. Depending on the type, sensors may employ a range of sensing elements. The range of an individual sensor may be as small as few centimeters to several meters depending on the power level, frequency of operation, and the operating environment.

Some of the applications are target field imaging, intrusion detection and surveillance, weather monitoring, detection of ambient conditions including those of patients, inventory control, and disaster management. Network of sensors can assist rescue operations by locating survivors, identify risky areas and making rescue team more aware of the overall situation in a disaster area. Sensors can be deployed either randomly such as dropped from an airplane in a disaster area or more commonly as manual such as installing on a patient's body.

4.5.1 Sensor Architecture

A sensor node has several components including those for sensing, processing, and transmission and position finding system and power unit (Figure 4.10). A network of sensors may have hundreds or thousands of sensor nodes, where each sensor can communicate with its neighbors or a base station. In general, more sensors lead to higher accuracy as averaging of more "sensed" values could cancel individual errors.

In a deployment scenario, sensor nodes can be placed in an area and co-ordinate among themselves to create highly accurate information about their surrounding environment. Here each node bases its decision on its mission, the information it currently has, and its knowledge of its computing, communications and energy resources. The potential of collaboration among sensors in data gathering and processing, and, co-ordination and management of the sensing activity can reduce energy inefficiencies, increase network lifetime and improve the usage of limited bandwidth.

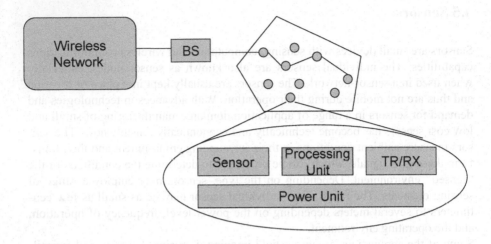

Fig. 4.10 The Basic Architecture of a Sensor Node

4.5.2 Routing in Sensor Networks

Routing in sensor networks is complex due to the large number of sensors, so IP (Internet Protocol) based routing is impossible as each sensor cannot be given an IP address. The other reasons are the energy, processing, and storage limitations of sensors. The other factors are the redundancy in sensed data which may affect which data should be routed and which one should not, and the presence of request-response traffic such as humidity > 80, which implies that sensors measuring the current humidity to be 80% or more should respond to the request. Other factors such as reliability, energy consumption, coverage, and data aggregation also make the routing in sensor networks more complex.

4.5.3 Sensors in Monitoring

Sensors can be implanted, on-the-body and be part of a wearable monitoring systems. The sensors should be low powered, miniature, easy to merge in their surroundings, identifiable, and reusable for maximizing their usefulness in wireless health monitoring environment. The sensors normally do not have much storage, so any application or device relying on sensors should store sensed information somewhere else for later analysis. Although sensors are considered reliable, more work is needed in ensuring that sensors are able to operate for long-term without requiring any service or repair. Since sensors are not mobile in their operation, these can form ad hoc or mesh networks to communicate sensed medical information towards the destination, including healthcare professionals. In many ways, sensors are considered front-end technologies that would require networking support for completing the monitoring process.

4.6 Radio Frequency Identification (RFID)

RFID uses wireless links to uniquely identify objects using dedicated short-range communications. When a product or person with an RFID tag enters the read zone of a reader, the address and data stored on the tag is read and can be sent to a server for location tracking purposes (Figure 4.11). There are two major types of RFID. One is passive systems with no power source, and where the tag's antenna captures radio power from a RFID reader, stores in a capacitor, and then uses this power to charge its circuits to execute commands and sends/scatters a signal carrying an answer or response on a different frequency. The second type of RFID is active systems with batteries, data storage, larger range and more sophisticated functions.

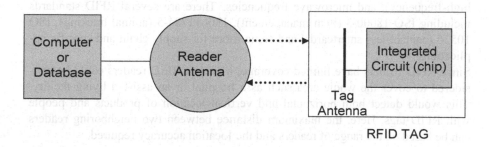

Fig. 4.11 RFID Reader and Tag

4.6.1 Use of RFID in Healthcare

RFID tags can be used in location tracking and identification of patients, devices, medications, instruments, and other health related objects. The tags could also be used to check if a certain medication or injection is authentic or fake. RFID is not an ideal tool for wireless health monitoring due to its limited memory and difficulty in periodically modifying the stored data. But RFID tags could store the identity and parts of medical records for its patient, which could be very helpful in emergency situations where a patient may not be able to communicate such information or healthcare professionals could not rely on patient-supplied information. RFID will not be deployed as a stand alone technology in wireless health monitoring, but will be a part of overall wireless infrastructure and can play a role in patient identification, tracking, and limited medical storage.

4.6.2 The Future

As the future identity theft may involve RFID tags, more recent advances include components for encryption, random number generation and key management. This increases the amount of energy the tag consumes and also increases the latency or delay and transaction times. Passive tags with security functions must stay longer than simple tags in the coverage of RFID readers. Active tags can support the security features easily due to their own battery. Some advanced RFID tags have anti-tamper capability, making them more secure.

With RFID, there are several types including those that are classified based on the frequency used such as LF (low frequency), HF (high-frequency), UHF (ultra-high-frequency), and microwave frequencies. There are several RFID standards including ISO 18000-3 (item management), ISO 11784-5 (animal tracking), ISO 10536 (contact-less smartcards) and some more for supply chain and specific applications.

Since RFID readers have limited coverage, a grid of RFID readers could be considered to cover the whole area such as a hospital or an assisted living facility. This would detect both horizontal and vertical location of products and people with RFID tags. Here, the maximum distance between two neighboring readers can be based on the range of readers and the location accuracy required.

4.7 Bluetooth

Personal area networks, such as Bluetooth, are designed for short-range wireless communications among computers, printers, cordless phones, and cell phones. Bluetooth is designed to replace wiring used among devices, so it is a low power wireless standard for connecting devices together in a small area. It supports data and voice and is a global specification for wireless connectivity. It uses frequency hopping at 2.4 GHz spectrum, so it may create possible interference from other 2.4 GHz transmission such as IEEE 802.11 wireless LANs, and microwave oven. Bluetooth allows the design of low power, small sized, and low cost radios that can be put in devices including toys, ATM machines, parking meters, vehicles, and clothing.

In Bluetooth, the basic unit of networking is piconet, which includes up to 8 active devices involving one master and 7 non-master devices. The total number of devices in a piconet can be as high as 255, but the maximum number of active devices is limited to 8. Multiple piconets could form and may overlap without any problems and such overlapped piconets are also known as scatternets (Figure 4.12). Some interference from oven & lighting devices and co-channel interference from other Bluetooth devices may exist. Bluetooth uses frequency hopping spread spectrum (FHSS) with 79 frequencies of 1 MHz each, where a frequency is used for 1/1600 of a second before "hopping" to the next frequency. Bluetooth packet has 72 bits of access code + 54 bits of packet header + 0-2745 bits of payload or data.

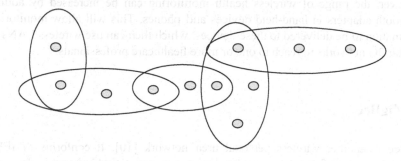

Fig. 4.12 Overlapping Piconets (or Scatternets) in Bluetooth

Bluetooth can be used in wireless patient monitoring as long as the requirements do not exceed the limitations, which include very short range, limited bit rate and not more than eight devices in a piconets. The range is about 1-100 meters for Bluetooth based on the level of power used. The bit rates offered are likely to be in few hundred Kbps. Both range and bit rates could be adequate for health monitoring applications, if frequency of monitoring is low with a few patients. For use of Bluetooth as an ad hoc network for patient monitoring, the limit of 8 devices per piconets would restrict the number of monitoring and other devices. This will affect the total number of patients that can be monitored. If multiple piconets are used, then interference in ISM band may limit the number of types of vital signs that can be transmitted for monitored patients. Also, Bluetooth enforces power control by dividing users among three types, which could affect the range of health monitoring.

In addition, there are many other issues that may also limit the use of Bluetooth for patient monitoring. These are possible crowding of ISM bands by the presence of other wireless LANs, interference from medical and other devices generating signals in ISM bands, and the usable capacity of ISM bands for transmitting a large number of vital signs for many patients frequently. Some of these issues can be somewhat alleviated by careful placement of other wireless networks that are not used for patient monitoring. It is also possible to use higher ISM bands or even a dedicated band for patient monitoring. The availability of a wider dedicated band will significantly improve both the quality and quantity of monitoring services for patients.

To improve some performance metrics, Bluetooth 2.0 has emerged. It is backward compatible with Bluetooth 1.0/1.1/1.2 and offers Enhanced Data Rate (EDR) of 3.0 Mbps. This 3-times faster transmission speed can still be used in 100 meters range. This could allow Bluetooth to be operated in multi-link scenarios due to more available bandwidth and the improved Bit Error Rate performance.

In general, Bluetooth is unlikely to be utilized as a stand alone technology in wireless patient monitoring due to its limited range and limit on number of users. However, the range of wireless health monitoring can be increased by adding Bluetooth adapters in hand-held devices and phones. This will allow monitoring information to be delivered to these devices, which then can use wireless LANs or cellular/3G networks to reach to one or more healthcare professionals.

4.8 ZigBee

ZigBee is another wireless personal area network [10]. It conforms to IEEE 802.15.4 standard for wireless personal area networks (WPANs) and is designed to be simpler and cheaper than other WPANs such as Bluetooth. It can operate in both ad hoc and mesh networking format. One of the intended environments is hospital care. It operates in the Industrial, Scientific and Medical bands, primarily in 2.4 GHz, but also in 800 and 900 bands in several countries [10]. There is also an extended version, called ZigBee Pro, finalized in 2007 for more features such as multicasting.

ZigBee intends to create an inexpensive, self-organizing mesh network that can be used for many different environments. There can be as many as 16 channels of 5MHz width in the 2.4 GHz band. The bit rate per channel is maxed at 250Kbps, but could be as low as 20Kbps in other bands. The range could be 10-75 meters depending on a range of factors.

It is more likely to be a front-end technology and will require another network to carry monitoring messages to one or more healthcare professionals.

4.9 Fixed Wireless and WiMAX

Fixed wireless includes wireless networks that do not provide support for mobility (or handoffs) but use wireless links for information transfer. One example is Wireless Local Loop (WLLs) that provides fixed wireless access. WLLs can provide several MHz of bandwidth that can be used for high-speed Internet access and data transfer in addition to the basic phone service. In developing world where installing millions of miles of copper is impractical, WLLs can provide phone and data transfer.

WiMAX (Worldwide Interoperability for Microwave Access) is a fixed wireless system, and it has been gaining some momentum. It is now an IEEE standard, called IEEE 802.16 and has five different versions a, b, c, d, and e. It offers high bit rates over medium distances. The frequencies are in 10-66 GHz (different in different countries, 2-3 GHz in US) for 802.16a, b, and c, while lower frequencies are chosen as 2-11 GHz for 802.11d and 802.11e. Many other worldwide standards are similar to WiMax such as WiBro (Korean standard used for cellphoneTV) will interoperate with 802.16e. Also, Europe has HIPERMAN as a similar standard to WiMax.

It should be noted that the advantages of WiMax or other fixed wireless networks are high bandwidth and metropolitan coverage (Figure 4.13). The limitations are lack of support for mobility, which may affect how patients could be monitored. The other limitation is the lack of availability in most places where patients may live.

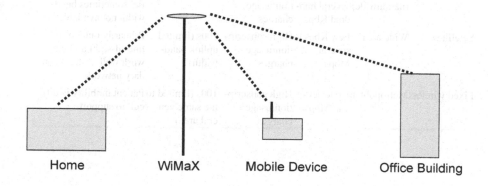

Home   WiMaX   Mobile Device   Office Building

Fig. 4.13 Use of High-speed Links in WiMAX in Metropolitan Areas

4.10 The Overall Picture

From a broader picture, mobile and wireless networks include several different types of networks as covered in this chapter. For each of these types, multiple standards exist today and the quality of service varies from location to location and from provider to provider. A comparison of many current and emerging networks for patient monitoring is shown in Table 4.4. It should be noted that most commercial networks such as cellular/3G, satellites, and fixed wireless will offer a high-level of security, while for networks such as wireless LANs and personal area networks more efforts are necessary to secure the healthcare information.

Table 4.4 A comparison of several wireless networks for patient monitoring

Wireless Technologies	Coverage	Bit rate	Cost	Number of patients	Suitability for patient monitoring
Personal Area Networks (Bluetooth)	Small (about 10meters)	Few hundred Kbps	Low with inexpensive adapters	A few (8 or less active per piconet)	Could work well in conjunction with other wireless networks
Wireless LANs (IEEE 802.11)	Small (about 100 meters)	Several Mbps	Low	10-100	Suitable for homes, assisted living, and nursing homes
Cellular/3G	Wide area (nationwide)	Few Kbps to several hundred Kbps	High subscription/usage charges	1000s	With commercial traffic, sometimes bandwidth not available
Satellites	Wide area	Few Kbps to several Mbps	High subscription/usage charges	100s (limited uplink bandwidth)	Primarily outdoor or line-of-sight and may work well as the secondary network
Fixed wireless	Metropolitan	Up to several Mbps	High subscription/usage charges	100s (limited to the same general area)	Patient mobility is difficult to support

4.11 Conclusions and the Future

In this chapter, several different types of wireless technologies and networks have been described. These include cellular networks, wireless LANs, satellites, sensors, RFID, Bluetooth, ZigBee and Fixed wireless networks. More specifically, a range of characteristics of different wireless networks are presented, and how their individual characteristics would affect their suitability for wireless patient monitoring is discussed. The wireless technologies are constantly under research, development and standardization. Many of the emerging technologies described in this chapter will be used in the future wireless health monitoring systems as stand-alone or in combination with other wireless technologies.

Questions:

1. Compare two different types of location management in cellular/3G networks.
2. Is there another way (except TDOA) to perform location management for E911. Discuss.
3. Discuss technical solutions to reduce/avoid interference in ISM band.
4. If you were designing a wireless LAN for healthcare, what will be the requirements? List.
5. What role do you see for satellites in wireless health monitoring?
6. In practice, if some sensors fail or go to sleep cycle, how will it affect routing of sensor information? Are there ways to improve reliability problems in sensors?
7. How is RFID different from sensors? Remember they both can store some user/sensed data.
8. How Bluetooth may be used in health monitoring? Discuss.
9. Draw a diagram to show the use of WiMax in health monitoring.
10. Make a table showing which networks use overlapping or same frequencies. Discuss the possibility of interference among these networks. Then recommend which networks can be used together in health monitoring.

References

[1] Varshney U, Vetter R (2000) Emerging wireless and mobile networks. Communications of the ACM, 43(6):73-81, June
[2] Dekleva S, Shim J, Varshney U, Knoerzer G (2007) Evolution and emerging issues in mobile wireless networks. Communications of the ACM, 50(6):38-43, June
[3] Guest Editorial (2004) M-health: beyond seamless mobility and global wireless healthcare connectivity. IEEE Transactions on IT in Biomedicine, 8(4):405-414, December
[4] Varshney U (2003) The status and future of 802.11-based WLANs. IEEE Computer, 36(6):102-105, June
[5] Varshney U (2007) Pervasive healthcare and wireless patient monitoring. ACM/Springer Journal on Mobile Networks and Applications (MONET), 12(2-3):113-127, March
[6] Varshney U, Sneha S (2006) Patient monitoring using ad hoc wireless networks: reliability and power management. IEEE Communications Magazine, 44(4): 49-55, April
[7] FCC Enhanced 911(www.fcc.gov/e911)
[8] Varshney U (2006) Patient monitoring using infrastructure-oriented wireless LANs. Int. J. on Electronic Healthcare, 2(2):149-163
[9] Varshney U (2006) Managing wireless health monitoring for patients with disabilities. IEEE IT Professional, 8(6):12-16, Nov.-Dec.
[10] Source of ZigBee (http://en.wikipedia.org/wiki/ZigBee)

Chapter 5 Wireless Health Monitoring: Requirements and Examples

Abstract Wireless health monitoring systems can be used to monitor patients' health anywhere anytime without affecting their daily lifestyle and to more effectively use the limited healthcare resources. In this chapter, we discuss the health monitoring environment, general monitoring requirements, vital signs, and some examples of health monitoring. We discuss how vital signs can be obtained and what specific vital signs can be used in detecting certain health conditions. Several examples are also presented, including monitoring of sleep apnea, arrhythmias, and stress. We conclude the chapter by identifying several possible monitoring types for the future work.

5.1 Introduction

The increasing cost of healthcare services, at 16% of Gross National Product (GNP) for U.S. [1], has created major challenges for healthcare providers, hospitals, insurance companies, policy makers and patients. Also, the number of people with physical and/or cognitive disabilities, currently at about 37 million in the U.S. [2], is expected to rise with aging of population. Health monitoring of patients has been proposed to reduce healthcare expenses by managing chronic conditions, resulting in fewer hospitalizations [3] and improving the patients' quality of life [4-9]. Further, wireless health monitoring (WHM) could support mobility of "monitored" patients and also of healthcare professionals, who can then be more efficiently utilized to perform other tasks and alerted only when certain changes occur in patients' conditions. Many more advantages of WHM are (a) keeping people at healthy level in their home or independent living, (b) delaying the transition to assisted living/nursing homes, and (c) an improved compliance to treatment and medications.

Wireless health monitoring systems would allow patients to be monitored at anytime in any location. Also, by using his/her medical history and current conditions, one or more actions can be taken including sending an alert message to the nearest ambulance or a healthcare professional. These services could use location-tracking capabilities of wireless networks including satellites (for outdoor tracking) and cellular/wireless LANs (indoor). Some level of intelligence (context awareness) can be built in pervasive services to avoid "false-positive" alerts, where an alert is generated without a real problem. One of the main goals of WHM is to reduce the time between the occurrence of an emergency and the arrival of needed help.

U. Varshney, *Pervasive Healthcare Computing: EMR/EHR, Wireless and Health Monitoring,*
DOI: 10.1007/978-1-4419-0215-3_5,
© Springer Science + Business Media, LLC 2009

Wireless health monitoring will also allow more un-obtrusive monitoring of a patient's chronic illnesses, and could obtain more realistic vital signs and biomedical parameters as patients conduct daily activities without being confined to beds or certain locations. Several health parameters, including weight, sleep patterns and activities, can be autonomously measured by embedding sensors in bed, toilet, bathtub, and kitchen appliances [10]. These will also improve decision making by healthcare professionals and eventually a better level of health and quality of life for patients.

The mobile monitoring devices could be implanted, portable, wearable or in the surrounding environment such as smart home. The devices with intelligence would detect certain conditions by the touch of a user. In the near future, many of the smaller medical devices can be integrated in the hand-held/wearable wireless device to measure pulse-rate, blood pressure, level of alcohol. In any case, a device would have sensors to measure a range of vital signs and other parameters for its patient.

There are several specific requirements of vital signs. This includes how to measure and process vital signs such as blood pressure (BP), ElectroCardioGram (ECG), temperature, and oxygen saturation. Each of these requires a different type of sensor(s) at a certain part of human body.

5.2 The Monitoring Environments

There is a huge diversity of patients that need to be monitored. These could include very active kids, who present a mobility challenge, where they may be running around all over the places and we have to make sure that portable/wearable monitoring devices still work properly and do not get detached. The independent adults may present a portability challenge, where they may not want to carry or wear a monitoring device all the time as they may say that they do not need these any more as symptoms are gone. For older frail seniors, we may have a usability challenge, where it will be difficult to put devices on their body due to their lack of strength and other limitations. Then there are paranoid people, who may present a trust challenge, where they may incorrectly believe that someone is watching them or trying to control their lives.

The types of patients, their chronic conditions and monitoring environment, and requirements are listed in Table 5.1. For each type of monitoring environment, including home, assisted living and nursing homes, several different constraints in terms of patients' abilities, closeness to a healthcare professional, and networking requirements are also identified in Table 5.2. We have also identified the most suitable wireless and mobile technologies for each of the monitoring environment.

Table 5.1. Diversity of Patients and Monitoring Environments

Patient type	Chronic Conditions	Environment	Requirements (what needs to be monitored and how)
Child and adolescent	Cancers, mental and neural disorders, pulmonary (asthma)	Home, Hospital or Mobile	Potential for very high level of "unpredictable" mobility
Adult	Cancers, hypertension, diabetes, stroke, mental disorders, heart diseases, pulmonary	Home, Office, Hospital or Mobile	High level of mobility
Geriatric	Cancers, hypertension, diabetes, stroke, mental disorders, heart diseases, pulmonary Falls	Home, Hospital, Mobile, Assisted living, or Nursing home	Low level of mobility

Table 5.2 Monitoring Scenarios and Requirements

Scenarios	Patient's cognitive and physical abilities	Location and mobility level	Closeness to a healthcare professional	Networking requirements	Suitable wireless technologies
Nursing Home (patient with chronic and terminal health problems)	Very limited (not able to interact with the monitoring system)	Restricted to the nursing home, slow mobility	Close (likely to be the same floor)	Autonomous Location-tracking in nursing home	Sensors, RFID, Bluetooth, ZigBee, wireless LANs
Assisted Living (patient with multiple chronic health problems)	Limited (intermittent and limited interaction with the monitoring system)	Restricted to the assisted living complex, slow to medium mobility	Somewhat close (likely to be the same complex)	Autonomous Location-tracking in assisted living	Sensors, RFID, Bluetooth, ZigBee, wireless LANs
Home care (patient with a few chronic health problems)	Somewhat limited (able to interact with the monitoring system)	Restricted to the home, but mobile in the neighborhood, medium mobility	Away (but likely to be the same area)	Location-tracking within home	Sensors, RFID, Bluetooth, ZigBee, wireless LANs, cellular/3G, satellites
Mobile Health (patient with a few mostly manageable chronic health problems)	Satisfactory (a high-degree of interaction with the monitoring system)	Mobile in the city/state, high mobility	Could be quite far (likely to be the same metropolitan area or state)	Location-tracking of the patient, services, and emergency vehicles	Sensors, RFID, Bluetooth, ZigBee, wireless LANs, cellular/3G, satellites

In addition, patient could be monitored in hospitals, which could include physical and mental rehabilitation facilities, long-term care, acute care, pediatric unit, neo-natal intensive care unit (NICU), peri-natal intensive care unit (PICU), coronary care unit (CCU), intensive care unit (ICU), emergency room (ER), operating room (OR), and medical surgical floors. These environments include very near-by healthcare professionals and their ability to deliver the needed healthcare services quickly, thus challenges of health monitoring are not the same as those involving patients in remote locations living their life as independently as possible.

5.3 General Monitoring Requirements

With an increasingly diverse healthcare environment, deriving and combining re-quirements of health monitoring involving fixed and mobile patients in indoor and outdoor environment is a difficult task. The general requirements of WHM are (a) reliability, (b) coverage, (c) real-time operation. More specific requirements of health monitoring can be presented and discussed (Table 5.3) under patient, net-work and healthcare professional categories.

Table 5.3.General Requirements of Health Monitoring

	Challenges	Comments
Patient-related	Vital signs (BP, Heart rate, Temperature, glucose level, Oxygen saturation, EKG)	The number and frequency of vital signs must be deter-mined
	Frequency of transmission (normal range, above or below normal, significantly above or below normal, high rate of change)	
	The number or size of devices	Each individual user may re-quire different size/type of devices
	Privacy and usability issues	
	Patients' preferences	
	Suitability for patients conditions	
Network-related	Interference and reliability of information trans-fer	Requires network infrastruc-ture to be dependable and available
	Formation of networks on and among patients	
	Routing of patient information	Requires complex routing protocols
	Performance (delay, traffic) issues	
	Scalability and network management issues	Requires sophisticated net-work management protocols

Healthcare professional-related	Number of patients per professional & cognitive overload	How much information can be routed to a healthcare professional must be resolved
	Training of healthcare professionals	
	Confidentiality and privacy of patient information	Complex legal and business challenges must be handled
	Liability issues	
	Cost and re-imbursements	

5.3.1 Patient-related Requirements

The health monitoring requirements include periodic transmission of routine vital signs and transmission of alerting signals when vital signs cross a threshold, patients cross a certain boundary, there is loss of contact between monitoring system and patients, or device battery drops below a level. These could include blood pressure, heart rate, temperature, ECG, and other health-related information.

Another major issue is how frequent monitoring of vital signs should be done. There is also an issue of what information needs to be sent and in what representation. The amount and the frequency of information that needs to be transmitted is another challenge. For some patients, depending on the conditions monitored, certain vital signs may have to be transmitted continuously, while for others periodic or event driven transmission may be sufficient. For all patients, any major changes in the vital signs should be transmitted immediately. Also, vital signs may be compared with some previous values to detect changes in values or patterns. In wireless environment, it may be desirable to transmit differential changes since the last time or a reference value to reduce the amount of information. This would also increase the chances of reception by others. However, the transmission of differential signals require additional processing by monitoring devices and the baseline values of vital signs used in processing must be known to all sides.

One of the major challenges is likely to be privacy. Here the patients may be concerned on who has access to the information collected from the monitoring process and how such information may be stored, analyzed, and used in the future. These are critical challenges and patients should be made aware of who has access to and what will be done with such information. The patients are likely to be comfortable with the notion of their caregivers, healthcare professionals, family members or designated friends as the only ones able to access such information. There is some evidence that patients, especially elderly, may not have much concern for privacy as shown by participants in a survey who did not believe that monitoring data would have any value for a malicious party [42].

As health monitoring by wireless and mobile networks include the use of wearable, portable or mobile devices, many usability issues including user comfort and trust must be addressed. Many patients including those suffering from mental illnesses is likely to make wireless health monitoring a challenge because of possible paranoia related to hand-held or wearable wireless devices. A level of trust from patients is also necessary for the success of health monitoring. An example of a difficult situation involves some people with mental illnesses that are inclined to think that some controlling entity is monitoring them all the time. Such patients are likely to be quite difficult in agreeing to be monitored by wireless networks. Other difficult cases could involve uncontrollable energetic, violent or frail people. The challenges are different as some of these patients will not allow any devices to be attached to them or may have serious doubts about the use of technology in general. Active involvement of healthcare professionals, caregivers and family members will be very helpful in convincing patients to wear or use monitoring systems.

The usability and portability of wearable devices for health monitoring must also be addressed to match the limitations and strength of the patients. Some care should also be taken to ensure that patients continue to wear or use the monitoring devices, do not remove on purpose, and do not damage the devices. Alerts can be generated if the devices are worn out, removed or are in no or loose contact with a patient.

Patient's preferences for monitoring technologies and how it is used is also important to the success of wireless health monitoring. A patient's current condition is also likely to be an important factor in such preferences and even in the ability to express those preferences. For example, people with dementia may need monitoring technology to have support for their decline in cognitive skills and poor recollection. The system may also need to provide them repetitive support for the same task. Some of the patient's preferences may have to be observed, if could not be stated by the elderly patient due to limitations. There has been some research on collecting patients' perspectives on monitoring technologies. Using patient interviews, the authors reported several key findings including their preferences for embedded sensor technology, some control over the system, simple interaction with the system, emergency use only, and stated that cost would play a major role in technology acceptance [42].

Also, the diversity of environments where patients may require monitoring and the variable length of monitoring such as short-term monitoring in hospitals and long-term monitoring in nursing homes must be addressed.

5.3.2 Network-related Requirements

The health monitoring will require comprehensive and high-speed access to wireless networks, reliable and scalable wireless infrastructure, secure and fast databases, and utilization of network intelligence and information.

The role of wireless and mobile technologies in emergency should support the detection of emergencies, emergencies notification, emergency vehicles and location tracking, emergency access to patient records, and support for delivering suitable healthcare. An increasing number of patients will be wearing portable or mobile devices that would have access to public or private wireless networks. To improve the quality and reliability of health monitoring, these devices could be designed to operate in ad hoc wireless mode also. With a lack of coverage and variable fluctuating coverage by infrastructure-oriented wireless networks in some spots combined with patients in locations not reachable by others, an increased reliability of monitoring and higher chances of transmission of alert signal can be achieved with the use of ad hoc wireless networks. Due to power and size requirements of these devices, the range of transmitted signal is likely to be small. Further, the range is likely to be affected both by the frequency of operation and the nature of spectrum used whether licensed or unlicensed. The range of transmitted signals by devices would affect whether or not patient's information reaches to a healthcare professional. For monitoring of patients who are not covered by an infrastructure-oriented wireless networks, the co-operation of others with wireless devices in an ad hoc configuration will be utilized.

If the networks are experiencing any failures, such as outages in cellular/3G networks or access point failures in wireless LANs, the monitoring devices could access other networks and healthcare professionals be notified who could then decide to use other ways to receive patient information. The last known condition may also be used in deciding or prioritizing the delivery of healthcare information. In some cases, patient information may be stored in the context-aware monitoring device and transmitted as soon as the network outage is over.

Health monitoring should include location-tracking where after a healthcare professional has received a message, the patient's location will be needed to send the necessary help. The health monitoring could include the use of one or more location tracking schemes including those using Global Positioning Satellite system. The user devices will be equipped with location-tracking functionality. The WHM solution should not necessarily be dependent on GPS due to one-way nature and poor indoor coverage from GPS and also due to the availability of several other location-tracking systems including Radio Frequency Identification (RFID). RFID can also play a role in differentiating a patient among multiple near-by patients.

The health monitoring solution should include interference and conflict management that could occur with flooding of user information. The use of priority can be used in deciding the transmission and reception order. The amount of traffic generated by WHM and the network's ability to carry this is an important requirement. The number of patients can be monitored is also very important. The monitoring delays and quality of monitoring will also decide the success or failure of WHM. Since most of the devices will have smaller battery, power conservation is important. In the end, WHM must be reliable as it is dealing with people's lives. Several requirements are shown in Figure 5.1.

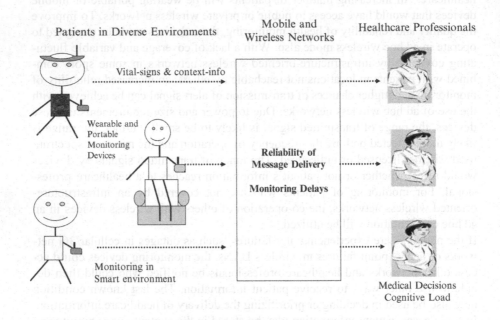

Patients in Diverse Environments

Mobile and
Wireless Networks

Healthcare Professionals

Vital-signs & context-info

Wearable and
Portable
Monitoring
Devices

Reliability of
Message Delivery

Monitoring Delays

Monitoring in
Smart environment

Medical Decisions
Cognitive Load

Fig. 5.1 Wireless Health monitoring

5.3.3 Healthcare Professionals-related Requirements

One major issue in health monitoring is the number of patients per healthcare professional and potential cognitive overload that may occur with frequent messages from health monitoring system. This is an important issue as the chances of medical mistakes could increase if a healthcare professional experiences cognitive overload.

Confidentiality & Privacy issues are important and must be addressed. The information from device to device will be encrypted in the proposed solution to achieve a certain level of privacy. In the near future, some work must also be done on addressing how to satisfy one or more provisions of HIPAA regulations on moving patient information from place to place.

Another important issue is that the proposed solution will create the possibility that a certain healthcare personnel could receive information on more patients than they are directly responsible for monitoring. It is very likely that the amount of information will increase, resulting in potential cognitive overload. More work is needed in identifying the increase in the information overload for healthcare personnel and ways to reduce it to a more acceptable level. The network routing could be modified to match patient information to a certain personnel using information from the database. There are also some issues related to liability if the personnel that received information about some one else's patient and did not take suitable action.

One major open issue is the total cost of the system. It is difficult to determine the total cost at this point, however a detailed cost-benefit study is needed that must include the cost of enhancing wireless devices with routing capabilities. The implementation and cost-sharing will differ substantially among different countries. For example, in the US, multiple wireless service providers, regulatory bodies, and insurance companies will be involved, while in many developing countries, a single entity such as the government could undertake the whole process. There may also be a need for additional training for system operators, healthcare professionals and patients.

5.4 Vital Signs and Medical Parameters

Worldwide, the number of people with a range of physical and/or cognitive disabilities has been growing. This includes about 37 million people in the US, or 14% of the population [2]. If the same percentage is applied to the World of 6.5 billion people, the number of people with one or more disabilities would be about 1 billion. About 40% of US seniors, or people 65 years and older, experience one or more forms of physical and/or cognitive disabilities, and with the aging of US population the number will grow even more significantly in the future. The same trend is expected worldwide as economies and healthcare develop and people live longer. Also, several million people in the US and other countries suffer from one or more chronic problems, including heart conditions, diabetes, kidney, lung problems, and mental illnesses. These people suffer from poor quality of life due to disabilities and/or chronic illnesses. The non-linear growth in the cost of managing disabilities and/or chronic conditions would eventually bankrupt any healthcare system, public or private.

One way to improve the quality of life for the patients, health monitoring can be used. The health monitoring involves measuring multiple parameters simultaneously over a long-term without disturbing the daily lives of the patients. Such monitoring can be facilitated by using health monitoring devices inside patients (implanted), over patients (wearable), near to patients (portable) and around patients (environmental). The examples are sensors, Smartshirt, hand-held devices, and smart environments such as smart house [7]. The sensors can be used as wearable, environmental, or a combination to measure a range of parameters. Wearable sensors are better for monitoring vital signs by attaching themselves on the patient's body directly or as a part of clothing (Figure 5.2). The sensors could form a body area network and may communicate directly or via a designated sensor to a device such as PDA or cell-phone, or may utilize some other network access. The requirements of wearable sensors are reliability, robustness, and durability; unobtrusive; able to identify users; communicate with other sensors and devices; and minimal maintenance and fault recovery [31]. In addition to vital signs, other health parameters can also be autonomously measured by embedding monitoring sensors in the patient's environment including bed, toilet, bathtub, kitchen appliances among others [10]. More specifically, these include use of sensors in bed to monitor sleep patterns, such as the number of positions changed in the night and using that to estimate the quality of sleep over a period of time. This could be used to help determining the quality of life a monitored patient is having and making suitable modifications including changes in medications and suggestions for lifestyle changes, such as increasing the physical activity level. A patient's weight can be measured daily by using sensors in the toilet [10] and bowl movements can be recorded for a later analysis. The level of general activity can also be monitored using sensors in appliances, doors, bed, floors, and individual rooms. Any marked decline in physical activity over a period can be an early sign of a more serious illness such as depression, which can seriously affect the overall quality of monitored patient along with the compliance to treatments of other chronic illnesses. For implementation purposes, a combination of sensors in both wearable as well as environmental conditions will be more practical to provide improved reliability of wireless health monitoring as well as comprehensive monitoring with more detailed information. There may be several different scenarios of wireless health monitoring, including monitoring by third parties for some fee paid by the patient/insurance companies.

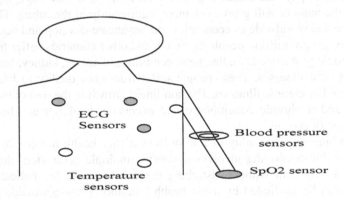

Fig. 5.2 Several Wearable Body Sensors

The monitoring system should operate autonomously without requiring intervention. It has been shown that health monitoring can reduce the number of readmissions for patients suffering from chronic health problems [3]. The monitoring can also help in keeping track of patients with one or more cognitive disabilities, such as the stray prevention system for elderly with dementia [11]. To support the long-term healthcare needs of the patients, while allowing them to remain mobile and not restricted to a bed, room, or tied to a location, comprehensive wireless health monitoring solutions must be developed for homes, nursing homes, and hospitals. These systems should measure several parameters, without affecting the daily lives of people, and the data should be transmitted to someone in real-time or near real-time. There are many challenges in designing and developing such systems, including diverse requirements of health monitoring, transmission of vital signs over limited and variable capacity wireless networks, and the medical decision making on the healthcare needs of the monitored patients. The comprehensive health monitoring system should also be context-aware, which will also aid in a better decision making by healthcare professionals on patient's current conditions and healthcare needs.

Wireless health monitoring involves measurement and digitization of vital signs, such as blood pressure (BP), Electrocardiogram (ECG), respiration rate, pulse, and oxygen saturation (SpO2), transmission of packets over wireless networks, and delivery of medical information to healthcare professionals (Figure 5.3). The monitoring system should transmit both routine vital signs and alerting signals when vital signs cross one or more "individualized" thresholds or match one of several undesirable patterns.

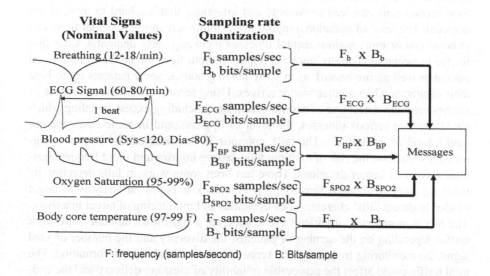

Fig. 5.3 Vital signs and processing in wireless health monitoring.

The nominal values of vital signs are represented in Table 5.4. The health monitoring devices [12-14] can be wearable or hand-held depending on the level of difficulty in use, portability, and the type of disability for the monitored patient. The device should operate autonomously and must send alarm signals when one or more problems arise. Once vital signs are obtained, these are sampled and digitized to group of bits before transmission in the network packets.

Table 5.4 Processing of Vital Signs and Parameters.

Vital Sign & Parameters	Sampling rate	Quantization	Total bit rate
Breathing rate	1 sample/sec	4 bits/sample	4 bps
ECG	240 samples/sec	12-36 bits/sample	2.9 to 8.7 Kbps
Blood Pressure	1 sample/minute	64 bits/sample	1 bps
Oxygen Saturation	1 sample/sec	16 bits/sample	16 bps
Core body temperature	1 sample/minute	16 bits/sample	0.3 bps

In addition to vital signs, the following patient parameters could be monitored: skin breakdowns, gait and balance (to reduce number of falls), motor activity, agitation, current location, cigarette smoke, and the amount of moisture in clothes. Skin breakdowns can lead to wounds and infections that are hard to treat, if not detected. The level of agitation, ranging from simple screaming to actual fight, can indicate one or more serious mental illnesses including early dementia. Checking for the presence of cigarette smoke is important both from the health of monitored patient as well as fire hazard, as in some nursing homes, some patients try to hide their cigarettes when a nurse/visitor arrives. Using sensors to measure moisture in clothes can help detect one of several conditions, including excess sweating which could indicate serious illnesses, the level of hygiene, and in some cases the patient's level of immobility. The falls, common in the disabled, are known to significantly increase the risk of multiple long-lasting injuries and more frequent hospitalizations of longer durations. There has been some work in falls detection by using an array of infrared sensors [15]. The work is based on analysis of target motion to detect falls' characteristics dynamics and monitoring of target inactivity. The health monitoring of patients could generate a significant amount of network traffic depending on the number of patients, the diversity and the number of vital signs, the monitoring frequency, and representation of healthcare information. The total traffic could affect the achievable reliability of message delivery and the end-to-end monitoring delay. The traffic generated by vital signs can be compressed, however, increased processing and packet delays, and, potential for "introduced" errors in healthcare information must be carefully considered.

The end-to-end performance in wireless health monitoring can be improved by transmitting minimal real-time information, such as differential signals or changes since the last transmission, over the wireless network and utilizing stored knowledge on patient and medical advances. Also, the comprehensive monitoring can be supported by allocating higher priorities for emergency and crisis management combined with pre-emptive capability to terminate non-urgent traffic over wireless networks. The health monitoring traffic can be managed at multiple places including at the source device, in the network, and at the health professional's device.

The vital signs, their nominal values, and frequencies and bits/samples are shown in Table 5.4. These values can be set as needed to accommodate more ECG leads, less frequent samples to reduce redundancy, and/or fewer bits per sample for different conditions and patients. In one of the monitoring prototypes [16], 250/sec frequency with 13 bits/sample resolution for ECG is found to be adequate for Arrhythmia detection. The WPM systems could also accommodate ECG compression [17, 18], with advances in compression and monitoring device technologies.

5.5 Specific Vital Signs

5.5.1 Measurements of ECG

The chronic diseases could become severe requiring medical attention, thus information must be prepared, transmitted and delivered to healthcare professionals for suitable decision on healthcare delivery. The severity of the conditions reflect in the changing values of vital signs such as pulse rate involving bradycardia (less than 60 pulse) and tachycardia (more than 100 pulse), blood pressure, breathing rates, oxygen saturation, and ECG. The basic architecture of the heart is shown in Figure 5.4(a) and a normal ECG signal in 5.4(b). Typically, when the blood is coming into any of the four chambers (right atrium, left atrium, right ventricle, and left ventricle), the chamber goes into relaxation (re-polarization) mode and when the blood needs to be pushed out, the chamber is in activation mode (depolarization). In an ECG signal, P wave represents the sequential activation of the right and left atria, QRS complex shows right and left ventricular activation, and ST-T wave is for ventricular re-polarization. The PR interval is the time interval from onset of atrial depolarization (P wave) to onset of ventricular depolarization (QRS complex) and the QT interval is the duration of ventricular depolarization and re-polarization [19].

The accuracy of ECG signal is influenced by the placement of different electrodes on human body. This becomes an even bigger challenge in wireless health monitoring where ECG signal is recorded with electrodes embedded in wearable clothing, usually for long-term monitoring. Both the location where sensors are placed and the degree of contact with body surface will affect the quality of ECG signal obtained, and eventually the correctness of medical decision making by healthcare professionals.

Although the use of smart clothing may allow an increased number of places where ECG can be obtained, work is needed in identifying optimal locations for electrode placement. A lead selection algorithm has been applied to identify the most suitable places in torso where the optimal ECG signal can be acquired [38].

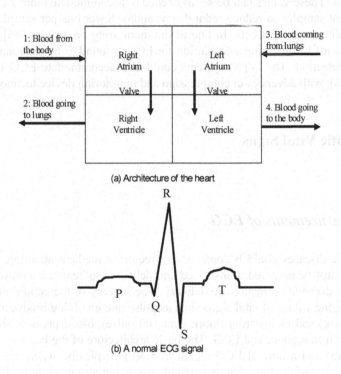

(a) Architecture of the heart

(b) A normal ECG signal

Fig. 5.4 Architecture of the Heart and a normal ECG signal

ECG interpretation normally involves looking at 5 different things: rate, rhythm (intervals), axis, hypertrophy and infarction [25]. The rate can be computed by measuring the length of a cycle over time. The rhythms are important as any problems in rhythms indicate arrhythmia. There has been some work in automated detection of QRS complex. However, a large variation in QRS complex along with the presence of noise affects the accuracy of automated algorithms. To address these, researchers have suggested the use of two or more automated algorithms to improve the overall accuracy. One such work involves an approach to automatically combine different QRS complex detection algorithms [36]. This allows the combined algorithm to benefit from the strengths of two methods. Additionally, the authors have introduced parameters, estimated by data, to balance the contribution of individual algorithms and have shown that the combined approach outperforms individual algorithms [36].

In general, any significant changes in wave pattern may indicate patient-specific cardio-vascular problems such as a missing or weaker P wave indicates atrial problems affecting the blood flow to the heart and a deformation in the Q wave represents some damage to the heart. A large increase in the Q wave with respect to overall QRS indicates myocardial infarction (heart attack), while inverted T wave indicates ischemia (or reduced supply of blood to the heart). A depressed ST segment indicates obstructions in the arteries [25]. There are many more such wave patterns indicating unusual problems. Most of the complex patterns and problems require comprehensive ECG signal using 12-leads, while simpler problems can be detected by signals obtained by 3-leads (Figure 5.5) [19]. These conditions could be detected by health monitoring devices (Figure 5.6). Also, some devices may perform a simple comparison of the current ECG signal with a prior ECG signal. And if there are significant and/or recognizable differences, it can generate an alert. More specifically, several of the above specific conditions can be checked by matching the above waves and/or segments before deciding what needs to be done.

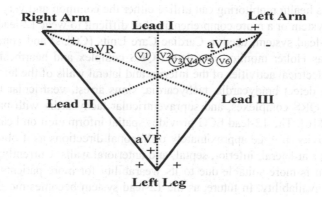

3-lead system = Leads I, II, and III
12-lead system = Lead I, II, and III, aVR, aVF, and aVL, and V1-V6

Fig. 5.5 The representation and placement of 3 and 12-leads ECG systems

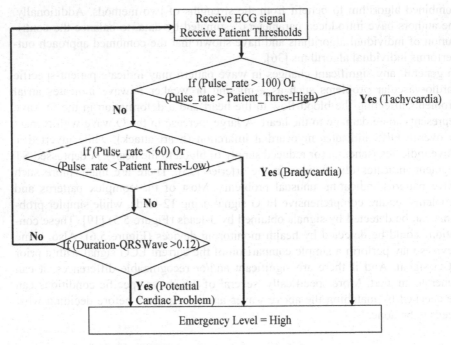

Fig. 5.6 Simple Analysis of ECG signal

The wireless health monitoring can utilize either the common and very popular 3-lead ECG system or a more comprehensive but difficult to wear 12-lead ECG system. The 3-lead system, used in Cardiac Care Units (CCUs) and commonly implemented as Holter monitor, can detect QRS complex and heartbeats as it observes the electrical activities of the inferior and lateral walls of the left ventricles. Thus it can detect bradycardia, tachycardia, sinus arrest, ventricular tachycardia with broad QRS complexes, and supraventricular tachycardia with narrow QRS complexes [16]. The 12-lead ECG provides spatial information on heart's electrical conductivity in three approximately orthogonal directions as it observes electrical activity at lateral, inferior, septal, and anterioral walls. Currently, the 3-lead ECG system is more suitable due to its wearability for more patients in nursing homes and availability. In future, as the 12-lead system becomes more integrated in wearable monitoring devices, wireless health monitoring can utilize it for a more precise and comprehensive detection of cardiac problems. To overcome the need for 12-lead ECG signal, some work has been done in collecting 3-lead signal and transforming it to 12-lead ECG signal for improved diagnosis. One such work includes the design of a mobile ECG trans-telephonic system [35]. A patient records and sends 3-lead ECG signal via a mobile phone to a care center, where a standard 12-lead ECG signal is numerically reconstructed using patient information [35]. The experimental study shows high accuracy of the reconstructed ECG. This will allow physicians and healthcare professionals to make much more accurate diagnosis in health monitoring. However, this should be compared with any errors introduced in the transformation of the 3-lead signal to the 12-lead signal and the additional complexity and processing requirements.

As the transmission of live ECG signals could result in bandwidth requirements that are especially difficult for wireless networks, the compression of ECG signal has been considered. One of the challenges is the compression algorithms that provide higher accuracy with higher compression ratio also generate higher delays and require considerable storage. This occurs as different frames have to be stored and compared against one another to generate an accurate differential signal. The delays may limit the real-time transmission of ECG signals needed for live monitoring of patients in homes, nursing homes and in remote areas. The storage requirement may also limit the type of monitoring devices that can be used in health monitoring. Some work has been done in addressing the delay requirements of accurate ECG compression and one example is based on wavelet transform-based ECG compression algorithm [37]. The low delays are achieved by reducing the frame size as much as possible while maintaining reconstructed signal quality. It also uses many enhancements including waveform partitioning, adaptive frame size adjustment, wavelet compression, flexible bit allocation, and header compression [37].

As some exercises could affect the load on heart, it is quite important to be able to monitor ECG signal when a remote patient is involved in an exercise. This could save lives as subjective abnormalities in ECG signal could be detected before an adverse event occurs. Also, very low heart beat or very high beat during the exercise could be associated with significantly increased risk of heart attacks. With increased availability of wearable sensors in different forms, collection and transmission of ECG signal during an exercise could become common place. There are some challenges including the quality of contact between wearable sensors and human body and the presence of noise affecting the quality of ECG signal. The movement due to exercise makes these challenges even more difficult. This could lead to presence of errors in ECG signal, thus affecting the overall quality of medical decision making. There has been some work in recovering R-R intervals, and thus heart rate, from such signals with unfiltered noise [41]. More specifically, a voting algorithm is employed to recover R-R intervals within a certain period. This allows for finding differences in ECG signal before, during and after exercise, but the output is not accurate enough to detect more specific problems [41].

There are several examples of commercial ECG monitoring, including CardioNet. The service known as mobile cardiac outpatient telemetry, utilizes 3-lead ECG monitor, worn either as a pendant around the neck or on a belt clip and a PDA like device which receives data from ECG monitor. If the PDA detects harmful changes, it sends the data to a monitoring center. The center could alert physician and calls the patient to go to a hospital. The device is used for 10-14 days to generate enough data to figure out the real problem as opposed to staying in the hospital for days [30]. Another system Medtronic offers is heart failure monitoring, which takes data from implanted devices such as pacemakers. The patient puts an antenna over his/her chest to pick up data on fluid buildup, ECG and other physiological data, and data related to pacemaker [30]. Another available product, Biotronik's Implanted cardioverter-defibrillator (ICD), can transmit heart information to wireless device such as cell phone, which can then send the information to a monitoring center for further analysis and action [30].

5.5.2 Measurement of Blood Pressure

In simple terms, cuff-based devices are used for measuring BP. These devices, based on oscillometric method, offer high precision and have been used in many health monitoring systems. These devices do restrict patient's mobility as the cuff inflation, which makes the arm immobile, is required to measure BP. There has been some progress in designing cuff-less BP monitoring using photoplethysmography (PPG). One implementation utilizes hydrostatic-based oscillometric method to create a compact, unobtrusive and low power sensor [34]. The PPG involves an optical signal related to the volumetric pulsations of blood, which in turn is related to arterial pressure pulsations [34]. The PPG sensor also requires a height sensor for measuring the hydrostatic pressure offset of the PPG relative to the heart [34]. The device can be worn at a finger base. Irrespective of how the blood pressure is measured, the values of blood pressure (both systolic and diastolic) can be compared with patient's normal range of blood pressures in deciding any abnormality or the level of emergency.

5.5.3 Measurement of Oxygen Saturation (SpO2)

Oxygen saturation is a measure of dissolved or carried oxygen in a medium, such as the blood. More precisely, it is the percentage of hemoglobin saturated with oxygen, which will affect the amount of light absorbed by hemoglobin in the blood. This principle is used in oximeters, which use red and infrared lights near to a finger or body part and measure the amount of light received by a sensor under the body part. The difference or the absorbed signal can be mapped to a SpO2 value. This also provides a plethysmographic signal, from which heart rate and further blood flow information can be derived [20]. Plethysmography is a set of noninvasive techniques for measuring volume changes in parts of the body, such as those caused by blood flow into vessels. A low level of SpO2 indicates several potential problems including respiratory problems, cardiac problems, specific sleep disorders such as sleep apnea, or problems with hemoglobin.

One implementation is HealthGear, a wearable wireless monitoring system, which uses a set of sensors connected by Bluetooth to cell-phones. It uses an oximeter to constantly monitor and analyze blood oxygen level (SpO2), heart rate and plethysmographic signal [26]. It uses Nonin's Flex Oximeter, suitable as light weight long-term monitoring of SpO2. Although designed for Sleep Apnea, HealthGear can be expanded to many other applications where SpO2 monitoring can assist in detection of one or more serious conditions.

Another major implementation involves the development of ring sensor for blood oxygen saturation monitoring [28]. The ring sensor is ambulatory, telemetric, and a continuous health-monitoring device. This wearable bio sensor combines miniaturized data acquisition features with photoplethysmographic (PPG) techniques. The ring sensor is capable of monitoring a patient's heart rate, oxygen saturation, and heart rate variability [28]. This can be used in many chronic cardiac and pulmonary illnesses.

As many sensors for SpO2 come in wearable formats including watch-type and ring-type, it may be appropriate to discuss which of these types may be more suitable. One way is to think that sensors should not be obvious to other people in order to protect the privacy of patients under health monitoring. Thus the size and shape of sensors, which may affect their prominence, may become important unless they match to current fashion or create a fashion of their own. A ring sensor may be camouflaged as a marriage or fashion ring, while a watch type sensor could easily be camouflaged as a regular watch or could be hidden under the shirt worn by patients. From the convenience part, some patients may be more comfortable with watch and some with ring. The patients could also choose one of the two options based on which one is more prone to removal both by daily activities and/or people wearing it. According to [28], ring is better for monitoring arterial flow using optoelectronic sensors and due to low weight and small size, rings are less likely to be removed than watches. In many cultures, rings are not removed at all, thus boosting the case for ring-type sensors in long-term monitoring.

5.5.4 All-in-one devices

We term the devices that can measure multiple vital signs and physiological parameters as "all-in-one" devices. These represent an integration of several advances in different type of sensors. On one hand, it is convenient to wear a single device as a watch, ring or smart clothing, but on the other hand, the functionality of individual sensors may not be able to meet some requirement. More specifically, if an "all-in-one" device uses a 1-lead ECG, it may not be able to produce the ECG signal needed for medical decision involving more complex problems such as arrhythmias.

One of the best examples of "all-in-one" devices is the advanced care and alert portable telemedical monitor (AMON) [27]. It is a wrist-worn system with sensors for BP, skin temperature, SpO2, and a 1-lead ECG, and an interface to a 12-lead ECG system. The skin temperature may not be a reliable estimate for body core temperature and 1-lead ECG may not be able to produce high quality ECG signal needed for complex medical decision making at the monitoring devices or by healthcare professionals. AMON contains 2-axis acceleration sensor for detecting the level of user activity and correlating it with the vital signs. The device can perform an analysis of all measurements and send to wearer and to remote location. It also uses algorithms to derive QRS width, RR distance and QT interval from the ECG signal, but in practice, the ECG results were found to be poor or not reliable as reliable heart rate or length of QRS interval was not possible [27]. Also, for blood pressure, diastolic pressure needed improved accuracy. Although the "all-in-one" devices are likely to improve in their accuracy with further technological advances, one direction may be the ability to re-program "all-in-one" device to "all-you-need" device for your problems. This focus on fewer vital signs needed for patients could lead to a higher reliability and lower power consumption.

Another major example of all-in-one devices is wearable health monitoring system (WEALTHY) [33]. This system uses a textile wearable interface implemented by integrating sensors, electrodes, and connections in a fabric form, and advanced signal processing techniques. The sensors, electrodes, and connections are realized with conductive and piezo-resistive yarns. These can measure respiration, ECG, activity and temperature. The system is suited for home/out-patient care of people recovering from an acute heart attack or those with chronic heart failure or an individual working under stressful environment alone. The ECG signal is sensed at 250 Hz, while respiration and movement activity come from piezoresistive sensors, sampled at 16 Hz. In addition, the system is able to process parameters in context, so that appropriate feedback can be given to the patient.

Another all-in-one example is the prototype of a wrist-worn integrated health monitoring device (WIHMD) with tele-reporting function for emergency telemedicine and home telecare for the elderly [32]. The WIHMD consists of six vital biosignal measuring modules including fall detector, a single-channel electrocardiogram, noninvasive blood pressure, pulse oximetry, respiration rate, and body surface temperature. The use of 1-lead ECG affects the quality of ECG signal. The device is designed to provide information on vital biosignals and locational information, with compromised fidelity to experts at a distance through the commercial cellular phone network [32].

5.6 An Example of Monitoring Scenario and Requirements

The example is designed for health monitoring services to the elderly in assisted living facilities or nursing homes. A brief description of such facilities, patients, and their medical history has been developed with the help of a clinical nursing home expert and also verified with recent literature on elderly, their common disorders, and quality of life challenges [21, 22]. This is applicable to assisted living facilities and nursing homes in the U.S. and modifiable for other countries. Also, the example, designed for patients with low mobility, can be expanded to cover mobile health environments with higher levels of patient mobility.

The patients in an assisted-living environment receive support from staff in daily activities such as cleaning and cooking, while in nursing-home environment they are completely dependent on nurses and other staff. The patients are involved in a few activities including getting ready in the morning, eating breakfast, watching TV in a group, eating lunch alone or in a group, sleeping, eating dinner, and going to sleep. They are visited by a nurse periodically and their prescription and non-prescription medicines are dispensed. The level of physical activity may range from no-activity to light walking for some patients, thus resulting in a low level of mobility. Multiple patients are assigned to a healthcare professional, however, in emergencies such assignments may change [23]. The medical history may include several inter-related cardiovascular and respiratory illnesses and illustrated in Table 5.5 [23, 24].

Coronary Artery Disease (CAD) is the narrowing or blockage of arteries that nourish the heart and is also known as coronary heart disease. The symptoms are Angina or chest pain, shortness of breath, arrhythmia, severe sweating [24]. Congestive Heart Failure (CHF) is when the heart can not pump enough blood to meet the body's oxygen demand. Usually a chronic disease, the symptoms are shortness of breath, fast/irregular heart-beat and edema in legs [24]. Acute Myocardial Infarction (AMI) is a total or near-total blockage of one of the coronary arteries that supply the heart with oxygen. The symptoms are pain/sweating, loss of heartbeats, and low to no breathing [24]. Cardiac Arrhythmias are disturbances or abnormality in the rhythm of the heartbeat and can be as simple as Bradycardia and Tachycardia to more complex ventricular tachycardia and ventricular fibrillation. The symptoms are major changes in heartbeats. Cardiomegaly is the enlargement of the heart. The symptoms are shortness of breath, irregular heart rhythms, palpitations and edema. Cardiomyopathy is a disease in which the heart muscle is enlarged, thickened or stiffened, reducing its ability to pump blood effectively. The symptoms are shortness of breath, irregular heartbeats, pain and swelling [24]. Chronic Obstructive Pulmonary Disease is an obstruction of the airways that progressively affects the ability to breathe. It is caused by chronic bronchitis or emphysema or a combination of both. Cigarette smoking is the primary cause. Symptoms are fever, shortness of breath, low blood oxygen, and cough/secretions.

Pulmonary Hypertension is abnormally high BP in the pulmonary artery. The right size of the heart gets enlarged and leads to heart failure and respiratory failure. The symptoms are shortness of breath, hyperventilation, cough and fainting. Pulmonary Embolism is the sudden blockage of an artery in the lung, usually by a blood clot. Symptoms are shortness of breath, weak pulse, chest pain and cough. Pulmonary Insufficiency is a breathing dysfunction resulting in the impairment of the Oxygen and Carbon-dioxide exchange required for body function. The symptoms are shortness of breath and reduced oxygen level [24].

The severity of these conditions reflect in the values of vital signs such as pulse rate involving bradycardia (pulse rate <60) and tachycardia (pulse rate >100). These vital signs must be processed, transmitted and delivered to healthcare professionals for suitable healthcare decisions.

Table 5.5 Illnesses, Symptoms, and Vital Signs of the Patients under Monitoring

	Illnesses/Conditions	Symptoms	Vital Signs & specific analysis
C A R D I O V A S C U L A R	Coronary Artery Disease (CAD)	Shortness of breath	Breathing rate (greater than 20)
		Irregular heartbeats (pain/sweating)	Irregular QRS complex and pulse in ECG
	Congestive Heart Failure (CHF)	Shortness of breath	Breathing rate (greater than 20)
		Fast/irregular heartbeats	Weak QRS complex in ECG
		Edema in legs	Low oxygen saturation (SpO2)
	Acute Myocardial Infarction (AMI)	Loss of heartbeats	Pulse rate (almost zero) and large increase in Q wave with respect to QRS in ECG
		No Breathing	
		Loss of blood oxygen	Breathing rate
		Pain/Sweating	Low oxygen saturation (SpO2)
	Cardiac Arrhythmias	Loss of heartbeat (in ventricular fibrillation)	Pulse rate (almost zero)
		Rapid heartbeats (in ventricular tachycardia)	Irregular QRS and high pulse rate in ECG
	Cardiomegaly	Shortness of breath	Breathing rate
		Irregular heart rhythms	Irregular QRS complex in ECG
		Palpitations (and edema)	Fast and variable pulse rate in ECG
	Cardiomyopathy	Shortness of breath	Breathing rate
		Irregular heartbeats	Irregular QRS complex in ECG
		Pain/Swelling	Low oxygen saturation (SpO2)
R E S P I R A T O R Y	Chronic Obstructive Pulmonary Disease	Fever	Core body temperature (>100)
		Shortness of breath	Breathing rate (greater than 20)
		Low blood oxygen	Low oxygen saturation (SpO2)
		Cough/secretions	
	Pulmonary Hypertension	Shortness of breath	Breathing rate (greater than 20)
		Chest Pain	Low oxygen saturation (SpO2)
		Cough/fainting	
	Pulmonary Embolism	Shortness of breath	Breathing rate (greater than 20)
		Weak pulse	Weak QRS complex in ECG
		Chest Pain and Cough	
	Pulmonary Insufficiency	Shortness of breath	Breathing rate (greater than 20)
		Reduced oxygen level	Low oxygen saturation (SpO2)

We utilized the services of a clinical expert, a medical doctor, who specializes in nursing home patients along with staffs of nursing homes in identifying wireless health monitoring requirements. Additionally, our requirements were supported by recent literature [21, 22]. Combining this with our observations and engineering expertise, the following requirements are generated.

- Monitoring of vital signs including pulse rate, blood pressure, temperature, ECG, and oxygen saturation for patients with cardiovascular and respiratory illnesses
- Monitoring in primarily indoor and some outdoor close to the facility
- Monitoring in an environment with limited and slow mobility
- Continuous monitoring, with battery power and physical restraints, lasting weeks or months based on the patients' chronic illnesses
- Periodic transmission of routine vital signs and transmission of alerting signals based on personalized thresholds or matching of one of several pre-defined set of patterns
- Very high reliability and low delays for alerting signal and high reliability for regular vital-signs

5.7 Sleep Apnea Monitoring

Sleep Apnea Syndrome is a group of sleep disorders involving repeated episodes when a sleeping person stops breathing [24]. This may be caused by a momentary blockage or obstruction in the throat or upper airway, or due to a dysfunction in the area of the brain that controls breathing. Snoring is the most common symptom of sleep apnea and may be associated with intermittent gasping, choking, and absence of breathing that awaken the person in a state of anxiety [24]. Episodes when breathing stops can last more than 10 seconds and can occur 60 times per hour and potentially hundreds of times in a night. These can be dangerous if the oxygen supply to the blood and brain decreases (while the CO_2 increases). Overtime, it can lead to headaches, debilitating sleepiness during daytime, and diminished mental ability and eventually, heart failure and pulmonary insufficiency can develop [24]. Sleep apnea can be tested by using polysomnography test, which monitors brain signals (EEG), heart beats (ECG), SpO2; eye, leg, and chest movement (EMG) among other things. But the test requires that the patient sleep overnight in a sleep lab or other designated location. There are three different types of sleep apneas. When the syndrome is determined to be caused by blockage in the throat and upper airways, lifestyle changes are suggested including increased exercise, weight-loss, and avoiding any sedating medications. But if sleep apnea is caused by a dysfunction in the section of the brain that controls breathing

[24], artificial breathing device is suggested. Also a dentist can design a custom device worn during sleep to reduce sleep apnea and snoring. If the lifestyle changes and procedures do not eliminate sleep apnea, continuous positive airway pressure (CPAP) is used, which delivers air under pressure from the nose to help maintain regular breathing during sleep.

Sleep apnea could be monitored with a variety of sensors and the information can then be transmitted to a healthcare professional. This will allow the patient to sleep at a location of his/her choice and monitoring over several days is possible. With this, the sleep apnea test is more reliable with patient being more relaxed sleeping in his/her place of comfort and night-to-night variations in sleep will not affect the reliability of the test.

One possible wireless monitoring of sleep apnea could involve monitoring some symptoms using sensors, then a longer-term monitoring of the life style changes made by the patient such as exercise, weight loss, sedatives and medications. The monitoring system would also allow the patient to enter symptoms and changes in life style made. This includes all the above that can be monitored using sensors such as exercise and weight, and also the ones that can not be monitored by sensors such as smoking, drinking, medications and tranquilizers. This could also be used to verify the patient's inputs with parameters directly measured by sensors. The monitoring system can send a reminder daily or whenever the patient is not following the changes suggested. This type of intervention can help patients in overcoming at least some types of sleep apnea.

5.8 Cardiac Arrhythmia Monitoring

Cardiac arrhythmias represent a group of conditions, where there is abnormal electrical activity in the heart, resulting in heart beating too fast, too slow or too irregularly. Some of the arrhythmias are minor and can occur frequently in almost all people, but some are dangerous and occur infrequently. These can cause sudden death for some people and can make others prone to a range of more serious problems including strokes. As the arrhythmias could be very infrequent, patients need to be monitored for a long period of time, which is not practical to do in a hospital due to the need for prolonged and costly hospitalization. Wireless monitoring is highly suited for patients who want to stay at homes, assisted living facilities or nursing homes. One or more of existing wireless networks such as commercial cellular networks, Bluetooth personal area network, wireless local area networks, or satellite networks in remote areas can be utilized for cardiac arrhythmia monitoring. Using sensors, patterns of electrical activities in the heart can predict arrhythmias.

One example of wireless monitoring of arrhythmia is Arrhythmia Monitoring System (AMS) [16]. The system collects 3-lead ECG information and combines it with GPS location, before transmitting over GPRS wireless network to a remote location. AMS uses a wearable server, or a data collection and communications device, which transmits information to a nearby central server using Bluetooth, which does data compression, location-awareness via GPS signals, and rudimentary arrhythmia detection [16]. Using the bio-sensors, 3-lead ECG signal is obtained, which can provide rudimentary beats and QRS interval that represents the contraction of both ventricles or strong part of the heart beat and is sufficient for arrhythmia detection. AMS uses R-R for beats, detection of bradycardia (<60), tachycardia (>100), sinus arrest when no atrial electrical activity for 3 seconds or more, ventricular tachycardia with broad QRS complexes when QRS>.12 seconds + beat>100, and supraventricular tachycardia with narrow QRS complexes when QRS<.12 seconds + beat>100 [16]. The system generates 22.5 Kbps traffic with 250 samples of uncompressed ECG and 13 bits/sample rate [16].

5.9 Wireless Stress Monitoring

Modern life along with our ambitions to achieve so much so quickly brings a high-level of stress to our bodies. Although some level of stress is necessary to be productive, consistently high levels and intense stress can lead to a variety of health problems and many self-destructive behaviors. When we are under stress, some changes in vital signs do occur. This could include an increased pulse rate, higher blood pressure, a higher breathing rate, increased blood flow to muscles, anxiety, and marked changes in the ECG signal. Wireless health monitoring system can measure some of the above changes by obtaining the current values using a variety of sensors and compare them to the nominal or at rest values of the person. Use of context-awareness will be very helpful to differentiate among stressful conditions from daily activities such as exercise. Then the wireless health monitoring system can send context-aware reminders to patients to slow down/adjust to a more relaxed activity. A long term monitoring over days or even weeks could lead to a more reliable detection of stress levels in the person's life and one or more interventions can be suggested and monitored for compliance.

One example of stress monitoring is the use of clothing-embedded transducers for ECG [29]. The system utilizes heart-rate-variability (HRV) to quantify stress level prior to and during stressful military training, and to predict stress resistance. The results indicated that the people who have better stress tolerance also exhibit different patterns of HRV, both before and during stress exposure. The Use of baseline HRV and the actual HRV monitored could be used to estimate the level of stress an individual is going through. Addressing this could reduce the probability of occurrence of any serious episodes including sudden heart attack or strokes [29].

5.10 Stray Prevention Monitoring

Patients with dementia, resulting in memory impairments, behavioral problems and other mental health challenges, are likely to stray when being outdoors. The significance of the problem is increasing with an increase in the number of older people, many of them suffering from dementia with aging. The development of a stray prevention system for elderly with dementia using Radio Frequency Identification (RFID), Global Positioning System (GPS), Global System for Mobile (GSM), and Geographic Information System (GIS) is presented in [11]. The residence sensor includes RFID reader to read patient's tags and GSM module for emergency communications. The body-attached rescue locator includes GPS module, GSM module, alarm, and human-machine interface. Four different types of monitoring, including indoor residence monitoring to detect if the person leaves a specific area or leaves home alone without notice, outdoor activity area monitoring to check if the person leaves a preset area, emergency rescue as indicated by the person himself/herself, and remote monitoring modes where family member to connect to the call center to know the current location, are supported. Family members or volunteer workers can identify the real-time positions of missing elderly using mobile phone or PDA [11].

5.11 Some More Types of Monitoring

In addition to several different types of monitoring as presented above, many more types of monitoring can be developed to assist different patients (Figure 5.7). These could include monitoring of behavior, medications, sleep and eating patterns. Certainly no single system could monitor all the conditions and not a certain patient would need to be monitored for all these conditions at anytime.

The monitoring of behavior is much more complex due to its difficult subjective nature and wide range of variations among patients. However, predicted/estimated behavior along with medication adherence, sleep and eating pattern could be used in detecting a range of mental health problems including cognitive disorders such as dementia. As medication adherence or compliance will affect the recovery from many illnesses and help manage chronic diseases, such monitoring will be very helpful to healthcare professionals and caregivers. A wide range of medical conditions can be inferred from sleep and sleep patterns. More specifically, information on rapid eye movement (REM) and other phases of sleep, along with number of times a person changes his position during sleep and leg movements, can be useful in finding out how well someone is sleeping. This information can also assist in prescribing or changing medications for the monitored patient.

Eating pattern is very important and ranges from binge eating, overeating, normal eating, and highly-restricted eating. The eating pattern has very different impact for different medical conditions. For some chronic and special diseases, the patients are restricted from eating certain foods, but should also eat a certain amount of food to manage their health. Overeating by choice or compulsion may lead to obesity, while binge eating followed by purging leads to another group of medical conditions. Certainly, monitoring of eating pattern may help obese and overweight people to loose weight and others to maintain their weight and health. On another extreme, a very interesting monitoring could involve wireless health monitoring of people suffering from weight and body-image disorders. This could include measuring symptoms of depression, anxiety, substance abuse, and more critically weight loss. Additionally, abnormal heart rhythm could be monitored.

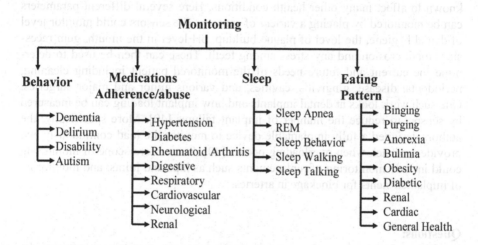

Fig. 5.7 Several Types of Monitoring

5.12 Conclusions and Future

Wireless health monitoring systems can be used to monitor patients' health anywhere anytime without affecting their daily lifestyle and also use the limited time of healthcare professionals more effectively. In this chapter, we discussed the monitoring environment, general monitoring requirements, vital signs, and some examples of WHM. We also presented several examples including monitoring of sleep apnea, arrhythmias, and stress.

Many more types of monitoring can be considered in future. Many of these monitoring types are for very specific and limited number of patients. Additionally, technological and medical limitations may have to be overcome before live monitoring of certain conditions become commonplace. The monitoring could include monitoring of transplanted organs such as kidney, lever, artificial heart & pacemakers, lung, cornea, pancreas, and intestine among others. The monitoring could involve collecting information on the functioning of transplanted organ, any signs of rejection from the body, patient's adherence to medications, and any prescribed diets and exercise regimen. Any activity in patient groups may also be monitored.

Another potential area of monitoring is in vivo pH monitoring [39]. This is useful in cancer diagnostics, diabetic patients and even trauma patients. With smart and miniaturized sensors which can be placed inside human body could communicate with small handheld devices.

Another promising area of monitoring is dental monitoring as dental health is known to affect many other health conditions. Here several different parameters can be monitored by placing a variety of sensors. The sensors could monitor level of dental hygiene, the level of plaque buildup, pH level in the mouth, gum recession, tooth erosion and any stress among teeth. These can then be used to determine the current and future needs of the monitored patient including cleaning, periodontal disease, gingivitis, cavities, and various minor and major surgeries. One such work looks at dental implants and how implant loading can be measured by sensors to reduce the number of implant failures [40]. More specifically, the authors designed a fully implantable device to monitor the load continuously and provide feedback when overloading occurs [40]. Some more scope of monitoring could include monitoring of replacements such as hips and joints, and monitoring of implanted stents for blockage in arteries.

Questions:
1. Discuss how actions of one monitoring components (patients, monitoring devices, networks, healthcare professional' devices, and healthcare professionals) affect the operation of others.
2. Are there any correlations among vital signs or are they completely independent? Why do we have to transmit all of them, why not just some and figure out the rest?
3. Compare 3-lead and 12-lead ECG systems on complexity, wear-ability, and usefulness.
4. What are the challenges in converting 3-lead ECG signal to 12-lead ECG signal? What specific patient information may be required for such transformation? Discuss any error that could occur in such transformation and compare that to the level of improved diagnosis possible due to 12-lead signal.
5. Discuss one type of chronic condition, where wireless health monitoring is most useful.
6. What is PPG? Can it measure both blood pressure and oxygen saturation?

7. Design a system to monitor transplanted organs. Derive what information needs to be collected and transmitted.

8. How is in vivo monitoring any different from outside the body monitoring? Can in vivo systems be reused?

References

[1] Kern S, Jaron D (2003) Healthcare technology, economics and policy: an evolving balance. IEEE Eng. Med Biol. Mag. 22(1): 16-19, Jan-Feb

[2] The website for aging and disability statistics: http://www.census.gov/Press-Release (March 2006)

[3] Toledo P, Jimenez S, Pozo F, Roca J, Alonso A, Hernandez C A telemedicine experience for chronic care in COPD. IEEE Transactions on IT in Biomedicine (in press)

[4] Stanford V (2002) Using pervasive computing to deliver elder care. IEEE Perv. Comp. 1(1): 10-13, Jan-March

[5] Boric-Lubecke O, Lubecke V (2002) Wireless House Calls: Using Communications Technology for Health Care and Monitoring", *IEEE Microwave Mag.* 43-48, Sept.

[6] Costlow T (2004) RFID monitors help trim health costs. IEEE Perv. Comp., 3(1):9, Jan.-March

[7] Stefanov D, Bien Z, Bang W (2004) The smart house for older persons and persons with physical disabilities: structure, technology, arrangements, and perspectives. IEEE Trans Neural Syst Rehabil Eng 12(2):228–250, June

[8] Jovanov E, Milenkovi A, Otto C, De Groen P, Johnson B, Warren S, Taibi G (2005) A WBAN system for ambulatory monitoring of physical activity and health status: applications and challenges. Proc. 27th Annu. Int. Conf. IEEE Eng. Med. Biol. Soc., 3810-3813

[9] Lymberis A (2003) Smart wearable systems for personalised health management: current R&D and future challenges. Proc. 25th Annu. Int. Conf. IEEE Eng. Med. Biol. Soc., 3716-3719

[10] Ogawa M, Togawa T (2003) The concept of home health monitoring. In Proc. of 5th International Workshop on Enterprise Networking and Computing in Healthcare Industry (Healthcom)

[11] Lin C, Chiu M, Hsiao C, Lee R, Tsai Y (2006) A wireless healthcare service system for elderly with dementia. IEEE Trans. Inf. Technol. Biomed, 10(2): 696-704, October

[12] Smart Shirt: http://www.gtwm.gatech.edu

[13] LifeShirt: http://www.vivometrics.com/site/system.html

[14] WelchAllyn   Monitoring   Devices: http://www.monitoring.welchallyn.com/products/wireless/

[15] Sixsmith A, Johnson N (2004) A smart sensor to detect the falls of the elderly. IEEE Pervasive Computing Magazine, pp 42–47, April–June

[16] Liszka K, Mackin M, Lichter M, York D, Pillai D, Rosenbaum D (2004) Keeping a beat on the heart. IEEE Pervasive Computing Magazine, pp 42–49, Oct–Dec

[17] Istepanian R, Petrosian A (2000) Optimal zonal wavelet-based ECG data compression for a mobile telecardiology system. IEEE Trans on IT in Biomedicine 4(3):200–211, Sept

[18] Al-Fahoum A (2006) Quality Assessment of ECG Compression Techniques Using a Wavelet-Based Diagnostic Measure. IEEE Trans on IT in Biomedicine 10(1):182–191

[19] http://library.med.utah.edu/kw/ecg/ecg_outline/Lesson1/index.html

[20] Battacharya J, Kanjibal P, Muralidhar V (2001) Analysis and characterization of photo-plethysmographic signal. IEEE Trans on Biomedical Engineering 48(1):5-11

[21] Spenko M, Yu H, Dubowsky S (2006) Robotic personal aids for mobility and monitoring for the elderly. IEEE Trans. Neu. Syst. Rehab. Eng., 14(3):344-351, Sept.

[22] Hauptmann A, Gao J, Yan R, Qi Y, Yang J, Wactlar H (2004) Automated analysis of nursing home observations. IEEE Perv. Comput. 15-21, April-June

[23] Several sessions with S. Varshney, MD on describing medical case and deriving wireless health monitoring requirements, 2004-2007

[24] AMA Concise Medical Encyclopedia, 2006.

[25] Primer   on   Basic   Concepts: http://www.fammed.wisc.edu/medstudent/pcc/ecg/rhythm_f.html

[26] Oliver N, Flores-Mangas F (2007) HealthGear: automatic sleep apnea detection and monitoring with a mobile phone. Journal of Communications, 2(2):1-9, March

[27] Anliker U, Ward J, Luckowicz P, et al (2004) AMON: A wearable multiparameter medical monitoring and alert system. IEEE Trans on IT in Biomedicine 8(4):415–427, Dec

[28] Asada H, Shaltis P, Reisner A, Rhee S, Hutchinson R (2003) Mobile monitoring with wearable photoplethysmographic biosensors. IEEE Eng Med Biol Mag, May–June, pp 28–40

[29] Jovanov E, O'Donnel A, Morgan A, Priddy B, Hormigo R (2002) Prolonged telemetric monitoring of heart rate variability using wireless intelligent sensors and a mobile gateway. In Proc. Second Joint IEEE EMBS/BMES Conference, 1875–1876

[30] Ross P (2004) Managing care through the air. IEEE Spectrum, December, pp 26–31

[31] Korhonen I, Parkka J, Gils M (2003) Health monitoring in the home of the future. IEEE Eng Med Biol Mag, pp 66–73, May–June

[32] Kang J, Yoo T, Kim H (2006) A wrist-worn integrated health monitoring instrument with a tele-reporting device for telemedicine and telecare. IEEE Trans. Instru. Measur. 55(5):1655-1661, Oct.

[33] Paradiso R, Loriga G, Taccini N (2005) A wearable health care system based on knitted integrated sensors. IEEE Transactions on IT in Biomedicine 9(3):337-344, Sept.

[34] Shaltis P, Reisner A, Asada H (2006) Wearable, cuff-less PPG-based blood pressure monitor with novel height sensor. Proc. 28th Annu. Int. Conf. IEEE Eng. Med. Biol. Soc., 908-911

[35] Hadzievski L, Bojovic B, Vukcevic V, Belicev P, Pavlovic S, Vasiljevic-Pokrajcic Z, Ostojic M (2004) A novel mobile transtelephonic system with synthesized 12-lead ECG. IEEE Transactions on IT in Biomedicine 8(4):428-438, Dec.

[36] Meyer C, Gavela J, Harris M (2006) Combining algorithms in automatic detection of QRS complexes in ECG signals. IEEE Transactions on IT in Biomedicine 10(3):468-475, July.

[37] Kim B, Yoo S, Lee M (2006) Wavelet-based low-delay ECG compression algorithm for continuous ECG transmission. IEEE Transactions on IT in Biomedicine 10(1):77-83, Jan.

[38] Finlay D, Nugent C, Donnelly M, McCullagh P, Black N (2008) Optimal electrocardiographic lead systems: practical scenarios in smart clothing and wearable health systems. IEEE Transactions on IT in Biomedicine 12(4):433-441, July.

[39] Korostynska O, Arshak K, Gill E, Arshak A (2008) Review Paper: Materials and Techniques for in vivo pH monitoring. IEEE Sensors Journal 8(1): 20-28, Jan.

[40] Van Ham J, Naert I, Puers R (2007) Design and packaging of a fully autonomous medical monitoring system for dental applications. IEEE Transactions on Circuits and Systems-Part I 54(1): 200-208, Jan.

[41] Cheng J, Jeng J, Chiang Z (2006) Heart rate measurement in the presence of noises. Proceedings of First International Conference on Pervasive Computing Technologies for Healthcare (IEEE), Nov.

[42] Steele R, Secombe C, Brookes W (2006) Using wireless sensor networks for aged care: the patient's perspective. Proceedings of First International Conference on Pervasive Computing Technologies for Healthcare (IEEE), Nov.

Chapter 6 Wireless Health Monitoring: State of the Art and Implementations

Abstract Wireless health monitoring has been an interesting area of research. In this chapter, we present and classify a vast majority of work done related to wireless health monitoring. This includes scenarios and visions, monitoring of vital signs, prototypes for specific conditions, monitoring for preventive care, monitoring for the elderly, and network infrastructure. We also present the evolution of health monitoring, a framework and an implementation of a wireless health monitoring system.

6.1 State-of-the Art in Wireless Health Monitoring

The current and emerging research in wireless health monitoring can be classified into multiple categories of (a) exploration, generation of requirements and scenarios, and future visions, (b) monitoring of vital signs and alerts, (c) design and development of sensors and prototypes for specific conditions, (d) monitoring for preventive care, (e) monitoring to support geriatric population, and (f) design and evaluation of network infrastructure for WHM. This does not represent all the work in wireless health monitoring, but our attempt is to showcase representative work from the published literature on wireless health monitoring and related areas.

6.1.1 Exploration, Requirements and Scenarios, and Visions

These are important as the exploration of scenarios and related requirements could lead to new avenues of research in wireless health monitoring. These could then be addressed by either the current technological solutions or by designing new ones. It should also be noted that not all identified scenarios generate immediate interests from research and development community or lead to practical and useful implementations. But these do push the horizon of the field and help people to think beyond existing applications, systems and technologies. A summary of research in this area is shown in Table 6.1.

The requirements of wireless health-monitoring system including diverse quality-of-service levels, context awareness, and network traffic management are presented in [18]. The intelligent monitoring is applied to patients with cognitive and/or physical disabilities, but have not been evaluated, tested, and implemented.

U. Varshney, *Pervasive Healthcare Computing: EMR/EHR, Wireless and Health Monitoring*, 119
DOI: 10.1007/978-1-4419-0215-3_6,
© Springer Science + Business Media, LLC 2009

Several requirements of continuous health monitoring systems, such as wearability, ease of use, affordability, re-configurability, interoperability, and scalability are presented in [31]. The general requirements of monitoring equipments are identified and a prototype for obtaining several physiological signals is presented in [8]. The work on deriving requirements for wireless health monitoring includes a requirement model for handling alert messages associated with medical tasks [16]. The alert monitor is designed to match medical staff and their mobile devices to receive alerts. The general requirements and analysis of wireless patient monitoring using wireless LANs are presented in [17]. This includes the use of wireless LANs for patient monitoring in several different scenarios, requirements analysis, and design of architectures.

Some usage models for health monitoring and technical requirements for the health-monitoring system based on wearable and ambient sensors are presented in [34]. The requirements of smart health wearable and several critical issues related to biomedical sensors, scenarios of use (linked to the business scenarios), data security and confidentiality, risk analysis, user interface, medical knowledge/decision support, dissemination, user acceptance and awareness, and business models are identified [3].

The use of protected, or licensed, frequency bands for telemetry will guard medical telemetry from the potential interference of other telemetry devices [23]. This could increase the probability of finding a telemetry product that provides the reliability, flexibility, and portability desired. A discussion of security and safety issues in medical environment, the technology, types, and characteristics of sensors, and research issues in smart antennas, denial of service, fault tolerant authentication, privacy issues, and energy considerations in patient rooms, clinics/wards, and hospitals, can be found in [36].

The use of standards-based technologies that facilitate the rapid assembly of wearable systems for patient monitoring is proposed in [38]. The component-based infrastructures allow monitoring systems to be configured 'on-the-fly'. The use of ultra-wideband (UWB) wireless sensors for continuous monitoring of health information is identified in [32].

In many ways, the work presented in this section may inspire future work in health monitoring. The requirements of monitoring can be included in the design of infrastructure and wireless health monitoring systems. These will also assist in how sensors and wearable monitoring systems are designed and utilized in the monitoring environments. The emergence of technologies such as UWB will also fuel the debate on whether to use specialized or general wireless technologies for health monitoring.

Table 6.1 Explorations, Scenarios, Requirements, and Future Visions

Focus	Details
General requirements of pa-	Diverse quality-of-service levels, context awareness, and traffic

tient monitoring [18]	management
Requirements of continuous health monitoring systems [31]	Wearability, ease of use, affordability, re-configurability, interoperability, and scalability
The general requirements of monitoring equipments [8]	Cost-effective, very rugged and safe for both the patient and the operator and configured for different parameters
Requirement model for handling alert messages [16]	Alert monitor matches medical staff and their mobile devices to receive alerts and rerouting of alert if not acknowledged in some time
Monitoring requirements using wireless LANs [17]	Wireless LANs for patient monitoring in different scenarios, requirements analysis, and design of architectures
Monitoring based on wearable and ambient sensors [34]	Some usage models for health monitoring and technical requirements
Requirements of smart health wearable [3]	Issues in biomedical sensors, data security and confidentiality, risk analysis, user interface, medical knowledge/decision support, user acceptance and awareness, and business models
Use of a licensed frequency band [23]	Will guard medical telemetry from the potential interference Improve the instrument reliability, flexibility, and portability
Sensors in healthcare [36]	Security and safety issues, sensors, and research issues in smart antennas, denial of service, fault tolerant authentication, privacy issues, and energy considerations
Standards-based technologies for WHM [38]	Will facilitate the rapid assembly of wearable systems and monitoring systems can be configured 'on-the-fly'
Use of UltraWideBand [32]	UWB Wireless sensors for continuous monitor health information

6.1.2 Supporting the Monitoring of Vital Signs and Alerts

In wireless health monitoring, the vital signs need to be obtained, either continuously or event driven, for monitoring of one or more health conditions. If the vital signs and other health parameters exceed certain "personalized" limits, an alert signal must be generated. The vital signs can be stored, compressed and transmitted as needed to healthcare professionals for medical decision making. Although, there is some debate on ECG as a vital sign, in this book we treat this as a vital sign due to its importance in several illnesses and the ability of monitoring systems to obtain and process ECG signals. A summary of research in this area is shown in Table 6.2.

A short range Bluetooth-based system for digitized ECGs collects short and long-term digitized ECGs together with relevant clinical data for the management of patients [24]. A design approach for ECG data compression for a mobile tele-cardiology model is presented. Authors achieved a significant compression ratio and reduction in transmission time over GSM network [28]. The development and implementation of ECG-blood pressure homecare tele-monitoring system is presented in [40]. This includes selection or design of devices to measure the vital signs. A wearable blood pressure monitor and the ECG amplifier were used to collect the data from these devices, process them, store them and feed them to a transmitter. The transmitter and receiver were used to wirelessly transmit and receive the vital sign data from the microcontroller to a personal computer at the receiving site [40]. A user-friendly graphical user interface using Visual Basic was developed to receive the incoming patient data from the receiver, store them, process them and present them in a clinically meaningful fashion to the health care professionals [40]. As part of European EPI-MEDICS project, a wearable, intelligent personal ECG monitor is used for the early detection of cardiac events [42]. It records pseudo-orthogonal 3-lead ECGs from an easy-to-wear 4-electrode subsystem embedding recording and processing capabilities, includes part of the patient electronic health record (EHR), embeds a web server and decision-making techniques, generates different alarm levels and forwards alarm messages to the relevant care providers by wireless communication [42].

Clothing-embedded transducers for measuring heart rate variability (HRV) and transmission to mobile gateway PDA are proposed [4]. This uses PDA as a mobile gateway to collect information from multiple sensors. The monitored signals then were transmitted to a central server using 802.11 wireless local area networks (LANs) or Bluetooth. The work showed the usefulness of HRV for stress monitoring. A prototype was developed to show proof of concepts for a specific set of patients [4]. Another study, using wireless LANs for in-home monitoring of heart-failure patients, included a prototype for monitoring of ECG and HRV signals from monitors to wireless receiver attached to a PC [5]. The wireless connectivity was limited to only between monitors and receivers.

A wearable healthcare assistant system, termed LifeMinder, synchronously records physiological information and contextual information. The prototype can sense pulse waves and user's actions/postures and captures contextual photos and continuous voice [27]. The context information could lead to more accurate alert generation and medical decision making. There are certainly major privacy challenges with such systems collecting detailed user information including pictures. There should be strict limits on how long this information will be stored and who can access such information. More work may also be needed to evaluate the trade-off between health benefits and potential for loss of privacy.

To support an alert mechanism in chronic care environment, mobile phones with Bluetooth communication capability are utilized by attaching these to chronic patients [9]. In this role-based intelligent mobile care system, an alert management mechanism in back-end healthcare center is used for emergency messages.

To overcome limitations of lower-layer wireless health monitoring, more work is needed in the upper-layers such as middleware and application layers. The use of middleware in wireless patient monitoring is demonstrated by employing wireless application protocol (WAP)-enabled phones in remote patient-monitoring and data retrieval [19]. The users could browse the patients' data, blood pressure (BP), and electrocardiogram (ECG) on WAP devices in a store-and-forward mode.

The use of intelligent multi-agents is presented, where each agent performs a specialized monitoring and diagnostic task. The agents are autonomous, interactive, mobile and capable of performing dynamic intelligent inference during execution. Decision functionality is demonstrated in preliminary prototype test cases involving emergency trauma scenarios, particularly focusing on stabilizing hemorrhagic shock [43]. This can be helpful in building more complex monitoring systems with agents as building blocks matching the specific requirements of monitoring.

A telemedicine system that can "bring" an expert specialist doctor to the site of the medical emergency, allow him/her to evaluate patient data, and issue directions to the emergency personnel on treatment procedures until the patient is brought to the hospital, is presented in [29].

The collection and processing of ECG signals by monitoring devices and subsequent transmission over wireless networks can lead to an improved decision making by healthcare professionals. With advances in sensors and wearable systems, the accuracy and details of obtained ECG signals will improve. Such improvement will positively affect the deployment and usage of wireless monitoring and telemedicine systems including those with for medical emergencies.

Table 6.2 Monitoring of Vital Signs and Alerts

Focus	Details
Digital ECG for patient management [24]	Bluetooth-based system for collecting short and long-term digitized ECGs together with relevant clinical data
ECG over GSM network [28]	Design approach for ECG data compression for a mobile tele-cardiology model. Authors achieved a significant compression ratio and reduction in transmission time over GSM network
Development and implementation of ECG-blood pressure homecare system [40]	Use of devices to measure the vital signs including a wearable blood pressure monitor. The information transmitted to a PC running a user-friendly graphical user interface for presenting the information in a clinically meaningful fashion to the health care professionals.
ECG monitoring for early detection of cardiac events by wireless communication [42]	A wearable, intelligent personal ECG monitor records pseudo-orthogonal 3-lead ECGs from a 4-electrode sub-system. The system contains part of the patient electronic health record, embeds a web server and decision-making techniques, generates different alarms and alerts by wireless communication
Use of heart rate variability (HRV) for stress monitoring [4]	Clothing-embedded transducers for measuring heart rate variability (HRV). PDA as a mobile gateway to collect information from multiple sensors. The monitored signals then were transmitted to a central server using 802.11 wireless local area networks (LANs) or Bluetooth.
Use of context information for better alert generation and medical decision making [27]	A wearable healthcare assistant system, termed LifeMinder, synchronously records physiological information and contextual information. The prototype can sense pulse waves and user's actions/postures and capture contextual photos and continuous voice
Middleware in wireless patient monitoring [19]	A middleware, or wireless application protocol (WAP), enabled phones used in remote patient-monitoring and data retrieval. The users browse the patients' data, blood pressure (BP), and electrocardiogram

	(ECG) on WAP devices in a store-and-forward mode (not real-time)
Intelligent agents in monitoring and diagnostic tasks [43]	The use of multi-agents, where each agent performs a specialized monitor and diagnostic task. The agents are autonomous, interactive, mo-bile and capable of performing dynamic intelligent inference during execution. Decision functionality in emergency trauma scenarios (stabilizing hemorrhagic shock)
Vital signs in telemedicine for emergencies [29]	Telemedicine system to "bring" a specialist doctor to the site of the medical emergency, to evaluate patient data, and issue directions to the emergency personnel on treatment procedures until the patient is brought to the hospital

6.1.3 Development of Sensors and Prototypes

The development of sensors and prototypes is very important from several different angles. One it shows that it is technologically feasible to develop such systems, second it shows the usefulness of some ideas for a specific condition or environment. Most of the work in this area is focused on specific conditions and will need additional work to expand its usefulness for other conditions. A summary of research in this area is shown in Table 6.3.

A mobile, low power, 32-channel, miniature, narrow band RF telemetry system (902-928 MHz) for real-time electroencephalography (EEG) epilepsy monitoring and evaluations is developed and medically tested [22]. The system enables several days of round-the-clock epilepsy monitoring while allowing the patient to be mobile in the vicinity of the receiver up to 150 ft away [22].

An ECG monitoring system for Arrhythmia is developed using Global Positioning Satellites (GPS) system and General Packet Radio Service (GPRS) wireless networks [7]. The monitoring system collects real-time electrocardiogram signals from a patient and combines with GPS location data before transmitting these to a remote station for display and monitoring. The system was designed for GPRS packet-switched wireless networks, which was only available in metropolitan areas, but now available in non-urban areas also. With the availability of EDGE, the system could be modified to support either or both wireless technologies.

Ambulatory monitoring is performed with wearable body area network (BAN) using off-the-shelf wireless sensors and ZigBee radio interface [2]. It uses accelerometers for motion and a bio-amplifier for electrocardiogram monitoring. The developed sensors can be expanded to monitor other physiological parameters [2] and also for continual health monitoring at home [15]. A wearable health monitoring system based on a textile wearable interface implemented by integrating sensors, electrodes, and connections in fabric form is presented in [35].

For monitoring of heart rate, oxygen saturation, and heart rate variability, a ring sensor has been developed for continuous monitoring. This sensor combines miniaturized data acquisition features with photoplethysmographic (PPG) techniques [6]. The ring sensor has been shown to be ambulatory, telemetric, and continuous health-monitoring device. One of the best examples of "all-in-one" devices is the advanced care and alert portable telemedical monitor (AMON) [21]. It is a wrist-worn system with sensors for BP, skin temperature, SpO2, and a 1-lead ECG, and an interface to 12-lead ECG. The skin temperature may not be a reliable estimate for body core temperature and 1-lead ECG may not be able to produce high quality ECG signal needed for medical decision making at the monitoring devices or by healthcare professionals. AMON contains 2-axis acceleration sensor for detecting the level of user activity and correlating it with the vital signs. The device can perform an analysis of all measurements and send to wearer and to remote location. It also uses algorithms to derive QRS width, RR distance and QT interval from the ECG signal, but in practice, the ECG results were found to be poor or not reliable as reliable heart rate or length of QRS interval was not possible [21]. Also, for blood pressure, diastolic pressure needed improved accuracy.

A new wearable stethoscope that is both wireless and battery-less is presented in [25]. The system consists of a sensor and a reader that uses inductive coupling as a method of transmitting the signals. This method enables the sensor to be free of wires and batteries, making it easy to attach to the skin. The transceiver antenna can be worn outside the clothes and the reader unit can be clipped on a belt. The system can be used to capture human body sounds such as respiratory sounds for the purpose of continuous monitoring of patients with asthma or other pulmonary diseases [25].

The development of a sensor to measure the alcohol concentration in the interstitial fluid (ISF) of a human subject is presented in [44]. ISF is extracted using vacuum pressure from micropores on the stratum corneum layer of the skin. The pores are created by focusing a near infrared laser on a layer of black die attached to the skin. This procedure for creating pores is essentially painless. Clinical studies show that the sensor readings are correlated with alcohol levels in blood and comparable to those collected using a breathalyzer. Alcohol could be detected in the subject's ISF within 15 minutes of the first oral intake of alcohol. Tests show that the sensor exhibits a linear response to alcohol concentrations in the range 0%–0.2%. The alcohol monitoring using the sensor was shown to continue even when the subject is asleep. The sensor is interfaced to a wireless health monitoring system that transfers sensor data over existing wide-area networks such as the Internet and a cellular phone network to enable real-time remote monitoring of subjects [44].

Application of UltraWideBand (UWB) technology to perform biomedical sensing and vital signs monitoring in humans is addressed in [46]. UWB is an emerging radio technology that uses very low power transmission for short range. The high bandwidth communications is achieved by using a wide spectrum, already assigned to others. The pulsed transmission from UWB would juts appear as low-level noise to transmissions in those licensed bands. UWB sensor could use radar principles to measure the heart beat rate and UWB communication standards to transmit these measurements. Several applications of UWB includes measuring cardiac volume, respiration movement detection and diagnostic, internal blood pressure, pregnancy monitoring, and monitoring of almost any object of adequate size such as vocal cords, lungs, and chest.

The use of Heart Rate Variability (HRV) to monitor response to stressful situations and as a marker for a variety of health conditions is also suggested [46].

As observed here, a significant research has been conducted to address specific conditions using sensors and prototypes. Some of these have been able to demonstrate the technical feasibility of systems to monitor complex conditions. These systems can be expanded to cover additional monitoring scenarios and conditions. The work in "all-in-one" devices is very promising, but needs to improve monitoring accuracy of some vital signs before such devices can be widely deployed in reliable wireless monitoring systems.

Table 6.3 Sensors and Prototypes for Specific Environment

Focus	Details
Real-time electroencephalography (EEG) epilepsy monitoring [22]	A mobile, low power, 32-channel, miniature, narrow band RF telemetry system (902-928 MHz) for real-time electroencephalography epilepsy monitoring and evaluations. Allows several days of epilepsy monitoring with patient in 150 feet range of the receiver.
ECG monitoring system for Arrhythmia using GPRS [7]	ECG monitoring system for Arrhythmia using Global Positioning Satellites (GPS) system and General Packet Radio Service (GPRS) wireless networks. Real-time electrocardiogram signals combined with GPS data before transmitting to a remote station for monitoring.
Ambulatory monitoring with wearable body area network (BAN) [2]	Ambulatory monitoring with wearable body area network (BAN) using off-the-shelf wireless sensors and ZigBee radio interface. Accelerometers for motion and bio-amplifier for electrocardiogram monitoring. The developed sensors to monitor other physiological parameters
Wearable health monitoring system [35]	A wearable health monitoring system based on a textile wearable interface implemented by integrating sensors, electrodes, and connections in fabric form
Ring sensor for continuous health-monitoring [6]	For monitoring of heart rate, oxygen saturation, and heart rate variability. Miniaturized data acquisition features with photoplethysmographic (PPG) techniques
Wrist-worn prototype Advanced care and alert portable telemedical monitor (AMON) [21]	"All-in-one" and wrist-worn prototype with sensors for BP, skin temperature, SpO2, and a 1-lead ECG, and an interface to 12-lead ECG. 2-axis acceleration sensor for detecting the level of user activity and correlating it with the vital signs.
Wireless and battery-less wearable stethoscope [25]	Consists of a sensor and a reader that uses inductive coupling as a method of transmitting the signals. The transceiver antenna can be worn outside the clothes and the reader unit can be clipped on a belt. To capture human body sounds such as respiratory sounds for monitoring of asthma or other pulmonary diseases
Monitoring of alcohol and transmission	Sensor to measure the alcohol concentration in the interstitial fluid (ISF) of humans. Sensor readings correlated with alcohol levels in blood. It exhibits

| over wireless network [44] | a linear response to alcohol concentrations in the range 0%–0.2%. The alcohol monitoring to continue even when the subject is asleep. The sensor is interfaced to a wireless health monitoring system. |
| UltraWideBand (UWB) technology for vital signs monitoring [46] | A UWB sensor to use radar principles to measure the heart beat rate and UWB communication standards to transmit these measurements. Applications in monitoring of almost any object of adequate size such as vocal cords, lungs, and chest. Also Heart Rate Variability (HRV) as response to stressful situations and as a marker for a variety of health conditions. |

6.1.4 Monitoring for Preventive Care

In addition to monitoring for chronic illnesses and/or generation of alerts for specific adverse conditions, health monitoring could also benefit in health maintenance or wellness for people without any chronic illnesses or health conditions. Primarily such monitoring would deal with activities, variety of exercises, health promotion tools and messages, caloric and dietary monitoring. These types of monitoring could also be performed for people with health problems as long as their prior conditions are included in the context and decision making. A summary of research in this area is shown in Table 6.4.

The monitoring and classification of daily activities could lead to reinforcement of healthy activities and eventually a healthier lifestyle. Several methods used for classification of everyday activities like walking, running, and cycling are described [51]. The focus was to find out how to recognize activities, which sensors are useful and what kind of signal processing and classification is required. Using collected sensor data from people with wearable sensors, daily activities such as walking, running and cycling, are classified using 82-86% accuracy. The authors propose to show "activity diary" to user to modify his/her behavior as part of behavioral feedback model [51]. Another study involved the implementation of a real-time classification system using a waist-mounted tri-axial accelerometer unit [52]. The system distinguishes between periods of activity and rest, recognizes the postural orientation of the wearer, detects events such as walking and falls, and provides an estimation of metabolic energy expenditure [52]. In a trial, an overall accuracy of 90.8% was achieved for normal daily activities, with higher accuracy for differentiating between being active and resting, postural identification, and fall detection [52].

The use of mobile phone as a health promotion tool has been explored [47]. A prototype application tracks the daily exercise activities of people carrying phones, using fluctuation in signal strength to estimate a user's movement. In a short-term study of the prototype that shared activity information amongst groups of friends, the authors found that awareness encouraged reflection on, and increased motivation for, daily activity [47].

The use of musical feedback to enhance exercise performance has been explored [48]. MPTrain, a system that users wear while exercising, has physiological sensors (heart rate and accelerometer) connected to a mobile phone carried by the user. It then assists the user in achieving the desired exercising goals by: (1) constantly monitoring his/her physiology (heart rate in number of beats per minute) and movement (speed in number of steps per minute); and (2) selecting and playing music (MP3s) with specific features that will guide him/her towards achieving the desired workout goals [48]. The authors found that the system (1) significantly improved the ability of runners to achieve the predefined workout goal, (2) made the experience more enjoyable and (3) increased the runners' perception of the workout's efficacy [48]. In future, musical feedback can also be applied to patients with a variety of impairments, including cognitive and depressive. When a device detects the patient doing, or intending to do, some recommended physical activity, it can encourage him/her by playing the suitable music. This could help in creating a better quality of life for the patient.

A mobile phone application that allows users to self-monitor caloric balance in real-time is presented in [49]. Termed, the Patient-Centered Assessment and Counseling Mobile Energy Balance (PmEB), it consists of a client application running on the user's mobile phone, a server application running on a web application server, and a web-interface that allows users to register and personalize the mobile client [49]. The server application sends reminder messages to the clients to update caloric information, stores the food and activity database, and keeps a record of the users' daily calorie data. The database is comprised of calorie amounts for 750 foods and calorie expenditure estimates for 37 physical activities, including values for different intensity levels personalized for a user [49]. A usability and preliminary feasibility study has also been done to show the usefulness over a paper-diary based system [49].

Dietary monitoring system could be very helpful for people going through restricted diets as well as for people, especially older, who need to eat a certain minimum amount for their own survival. Dietary monitoring includes a variety of aspects such as timing and frequency of eating activities, rate of intake as well as type and amount of foodstuff. One way to design such system is to consider swallowing detection as swallowing is inherently linked to eating and drinking activities [50]. The detection and classification targets the analysis of pharyngeal swallowing using non-invasive sensors attached to the user's neck. The overall concept relates to the problems of sensor data acquisition, event detection and classification. The authors present an investigation to detect and classify normal swallowing during eating and drinking from electromyography and microphone sensors [50]. The non-invasive sensors are selected in order to integrate them into a collar-like fabric for continuous monitoring of swallowing activity over a day. The authors compare methods for the detection of individual swallowing events from continuous sensor data. The methods are evaluated on experimental data and a performance analysis shows a level of accuracy [50]. The swallowing detection systems can be expanded to detect any object that a baby may have swallowed and create an alarm accordingly for the caregiver or family member. More specifically, babies normally eat liquid or semi-solid food for the first 1-2 years of their life and the systems can detect any solid object or food the baby under monitoring may have eaten [50].

As part of preventive care, one promising area is healthy aging. One such work focuses on using consumer electronic devices to motivate healthy behavior by presenting information at points of decision and behavior [55]. These devices could provide motivational health messages or feedback tailored to individuals at the right time at the right places to choose healthy behavior including exercise and healthy diets [55]. The author suggests that longitudinal feedback, without aggravating the user, could lead to slow and steady behavior changes to improve quality of life and overall health [55].

The work in this section is very promising as it focuses on monitoring of conditions that could lead to healthier life styles and support preventive care. The work here includes monitoring of daily activities, sharing the information of activities among friends, musical feedback, caloric monitoring and swallowing detection. These advances, using technical, social and human characteristics could be combined into one system for improving general wellness. The improvement in the quality of life and long-term reduction in the healthcare cost could be enormous.

Table 6.4 Monitoring for Preventive Care

Focus	Details
Monitoring and classification of daily activities for healthier lifestyle [51]	The monitoring and classification of daily activities for reinforcement of healthy activities and eventually a healthier lifestyle. Using collected data from wearable sensors, daily activities such as walking, running and cycling, are classified at 82-86% accuracy and shown to users to modify behavior
Tracking user activity and sharing among users for increased motivation [47]	Mobile phone as a health promotion tool, where an application tracks the daily exercise activities of people carrying phones (fluctuation in signal strength to estimate movement). Sharing of activity information amongst groups of friends increased motivation for daily activity.
Musical feedback to enhance exercise performance [48]	MPTrain, a wearable system with physiological sensors (heart rate and accelerometer) connected to a mobile phone. It helps in achieving the desired exercising goals by: constantly monitoring heart beats per minute and movement and selecting and playing music (MP3s) with specific features to help workout goals.
Self-monitoring of caloric balance in real-time [49]	Mobile application to allow users to self-monitor caloric balance in real-time. The server application asks the clients to update caloric information, stores the food and activity database, and keeps daily calorie data. More useful than a paper-diary based system.
Swallowing detection using sensors [50]	Dietary monitoring: timing and frequency of eating activities, rate of intake as well as type and amount of foodstuff. Analysis of pharyngeal swallowing using non-invasive sensors at user's neck (collar-like fabric). Detection and classification of normal swallowing during eating and drinking from electromyography and microphone sensors.

Healthy aging by using motivational messages from devices [55]	Use of consumer electronic devices to motivate healthy behavior by presenting information at points of decision and behavior. These devices provide motivational health messages or feedback tailored to individuals at the right time at the right places to choose healthy behavior including exercise and healthy diet.

6.1.5 Monitoring to Support Geriatric Population

One of the goals of monitoring technologies for geriatric population is to allow them to stay, independently at homes, or with some support at assisted living facilities. Many technologies attempt to at least delay their transition to nursing homes, where there is very little independence for older people. It has been known for some time that older people are open to, and even interested in learning, a range of wireless technologies to help keeping them at their home independently. The growing percentage of elderly people in society calls for novel healthcare support services to enhance elders' daily life independence in indoor and outdoor environments [33]. The support for geriatric population is one of the most promising for WHM due to both the number of chronic conditions and the sheer number of patients, expected to grow even higher in the near future. One of the most promising areas is fall prevention and detection. A large number of hospitalization for geriatric patients result due to complications caused by falls. The use of wireless technologies to reduce the number of falls as well as detecting falls and getting immediate help can save billions of dollars per year. A range of sensors, positioning and related technologies are under development to address this need of older patients. A summary of research in this area is shown in Table 6.5.

One broad set of implementations involve smart home or smart house, where different technologies are embedded to help them in their daily activities. A detailed overview of smart house for older and/or disabled people including wireless patient monitoring systems can be found in [1]. Another prototype for elderly includes a wrist-worn integrated health monitoring device (WIHMD) with six modules for fall detection, electrocardiogram, blood pressure, pulse oximetry, respiration rate, and body temperature [13]. It uses cellular phone network for transmission of vital bio-signals and locational information to experts at a distance through the commercial cellular phone network.

Another monitoring system for elderly involves an implementation using wireless channels and wired LANs in nursing homes [11]. Additional work for monitoring of elderly includes development of two rehabilitation devices, or personal aids for mobility and monitoring [12]. The aids are shown to provide support, guidance, and health monitoring in an assisted living facility. The devices are intended to delay the transition from eldercare or assisted living facilities to nursing homes. The robotic PAMMs provide support, guidance, and health monitoring. Two experimental systems and experimental data from trials in an assisted living facility using both systems are presented [12].

Prototyping of wireless patient monitoring systems that focus on elderly includes a stray prevention system for elderly with dementia using Radio Frequency Identification (RFID), GPS, Global System for Mobile (GSM) and Geographical Information Systems (GIS) [10]. Four different types of monitoring, indoor residence monitoring, outdoor activity area monitoring, emergency rescue, and remote monitoring modes, are supported. Family members or volunteer workers can identify the real-time positions of missing elderly using mobile phone or PDA.

With increasing dementia, many elderly have difficulty in conducting day to day life activities. This could even involve simple activities such as brushing, showering, and hand-washing. To help the elderly with dementia, caregivers may have to assist them in completing such activities. Automated systems could be designed to reduce such reliance on caregivers and also reduce the level of frustration when immediate help from caregivers is not available. There has been some work in designing and evaluating such system, which uses Markov decision processes (MDPs) to determine when and how to provide prompts to a user with dementia for guidance through the activity of hand-washing [53]. This work could be expanded to cover other daily activities and future guidance systems could be designed.

Monitoring of daily activities of people living in assisted-living facilities can be used in detecting potential health problems and informing caregivers and healthcare professionals. Some work has been done in collecting behavioral patterns from activity monitoring of people in assisted-living facilities [56]. Using a predictive algorithm that models circadian (daily) activity rhythms, consisting of the average time a resident spent in each room and the number of motion events per room, and their deviations, established behavioral patterns are obtained [56]. Using the deviations from activity rhythms, some changes in health conditions could be predicted and caregivers and healthcare professionals could be informed.

One of the most suitable targets for wireless health monitoring is likely to be the growing geriatric population. The elderly people want to live as independently as possible, while remain connected with friends and family members, and are likely to accept wireless technologies to support their daily activities and healthcare monitoring. Certainly, much more work is needed in matching the technologies to the patients' needs and capabilities, and understanding the acceptance and usage of wireless technology among geriatric population. The different roles of healthcare professionals, caregivers, family members and friends in helping geriatric patients to adopt monitoring and assistive technologies can also be explored.

Table 6.5 Monitoring for Geriatric Population

Focus	Details
A detailed overview of	One broad set of implementations involve smart home/house, where

smart house for older or disabled people [1]	different technologies are embedded to help them in their daily activities. This includes wireless patient monitoring systems.
Wrist-worn integrated health monitoring device (WIHMD) [13]	WIHMD with six modules for fall detection, electrocardiogram, blood pressure, pulse oximetry, respiration rate, and body temperature. Cellular phone network for transmission of vital bio-signals and locational information with compromised fidelity to experts at a distance
Wireless monitoring system for elderly [11]	Wireless monitoring system for elderly using wireless channels and wired LANs in nursing homes
Personal aids for mobility and monitoring (PAMMs) [12]	Development of two rehabilitation devices. The robotic aids provide support, guidance, and health monitoring. Experimental data from trials in an assisted living
Monitoring and stray prevention system for elderly with dementia [10]	Prototyping of WHM using RFID, GPS, GSM and Geographical Information Systems (GIS). Family members or volunteer identify the real-time positions of missing elderly using mobile phone or PDA.
Guidance system for elderly [53]	The use of Markov decision processes (MDPs) to determine when and how to provide prompts to a user with dementia for guidance through the activity of hand-washing.
Monitoring of deviations from daily rhythms to predict health changes [56]	Using a predictive algorithm that models circadian (daily) activity rhythms and their deviations, established behavioral patterns are obtained. Using the deviations from activity rhythms, changes in health conditions predicted and healthcare professionals informed.

6.1.6 Network Infrastructure for WHM

The networking infrastructure must support transmission of vital signs and related information to one or more healthcare professionals, who may be far way from the monitored patients. The range of networks could be as small as body area connecting sensors on patient's body to satellite networks covering much larger distances. Wireless LANs and commercial cellular networks are used for distances in between. The work in this area includes both the application of existing networks to support health monitoring as well as designing new networks to address coverage, reliability and limited power challenges. A summary of research in this area is shown in Table 6.6.

A method for making wireless body-worn medical sensors aware of the persons they belong to by combining body-coupled with wireless communication is presented in [45]. This enables a user to create a wireless body sensor network by just sticking the sensors to her body. A personal identifier allows sensors to annotate their readings with a user ID thereby ensuring safety in personal healthcare environments with multiple users [45]. This is important for both the integrity and security of data. The data security should ensure that the information is coming from the intended person, is being processed by intended equipment, and will go to the correct healthcare professional.

A portable parameter monitoring and analysis system for physiological studies for assisting patient-centric health care management is developed [41]. The system uses network approach to acquire the data from sensors and transmit the data on to a server through wireless means. The system automates the acquisition of physiological parameters by continuous display on the monitor screen [41].

The use of Bluetooth and wireless LANs has been proposed with four different monitoring devices to meet the requirements of medical personnel [14]. The design of a processor, which samples signals from sensors on the patient, is presented in [30]. It then transmits digital data over a Bluetooth link to a mobile telephone that uses the General Packet Radio Service. An integration of sensors and actuators to a Wireless Body Area Network (BAN), followed by 2.5 (GPRS) and 3G (UMTS) technologies is proposed in [39]. These sensors and actuators continuously measure and transmit vital constants along with voice and images/video to health service providers. Remote assistance in case of accidents is provided by allowing the paramedics to send reliable vital constants data as well as audio and video directly from the accident site [39].

To support the quality of service (QoS) requirements for medical calls, mobile sensor networks and 3G cellular networks are used [20]. The work involves the use of a low-energy, distributed, and data query mechanism that uses hierarchical ad hoc routing algorithms to enable a medical specialist to collect physiological data from mobile and/or remote patients. The medical specialist uses cellular network to report patients' data to the medical center [20]. The work needs extensions to make it suitable for wireless health monitoring.

The Future Home project has focused on specifying and implementing a wireless residential networking and gateway system. The main objective is the integration of heterogeneous wireless technologies, IPv6, and middleware for services. The authors provide a description of the future home technological concept and results from the user interviews about their opinions on different health related scenarios [37].

The use of ad hoc networks to supplement infrastructure-oriented wireless networks for health monitoring has been proposed. As part of providing reliability with power conservation, power management protocols and sleep cycles are presented in [26].

As most cellular networks are designed around capacity for voice traffic, some work has been done in addressing the future design of wireless networks for data traffic requirements of healthcare. A proposed design for 3G networks using coverage and capacity constraints has been presented [54]. The authors have shown that strategic placement of base stations could satisfy both coverage and data capacity for healthcare applications [54].

As it can be observed that several different choices of infrastructure may exist for wireless health monitoring. More work is needed in demonstrating the level of reliability needed for health monitoring, the level of integration and interoperability among different infrastructure, and the quality of service support in wireless networks for health monitoring.

Table 6.6 Design and Evaluation of Network Infrastructure

Focus	Details
Creating user identification in medical sensors [45]	Making wireless body-worn medical sensors aware of the persons they belong to by combining body with wireless communication. A personal identifier allows sensors to annotate their readings with a user ID thereby ensuring safety in personal healthcare environments with multiple users.
Transmitting from sensors to a GPRS phone [30]	The processor samples signals from sensors on the patient, then transmits digital data over a Bluetooth link to a mobile telephone that uses the General Packet Radio Service.
An integration of sensors to a Wireless Body Area Network (BAN), followed by GPRS and 3G [39]	An integration of sensors and actuators to a Wireless Body Area Network (BAN), followed by 2.5 (GPRS) and 3G (UMTS) technologies. These sensors and actuators continuously measure and transmit vital constants along with voice and images/video to health service providers. Also useful for remote assistance in case of accidents
Quality of service (QoS) requirements for medical calls, mobile sensor networks and 3G cellular networks [20]	To support the quality of service (QoS) requirements for medical calls, mobile sensor networks and 3G cellular networks are used. Use of a data query mechanism to enable a medical specialist to collect physiological data from remote patients. The specialist uses cellular network to report patients' data to the medical center.
The Future Home [37]	Focused on specifying and implementing a wireless residential networking and gateway system. Integration of heterogeneous wireless technologies, IPv6, and middleware for services. A description of the future home technological concept and results from the user interviews on different health related scenarios
Use of ad hoc networks to supplement infrastructure-oriented wireless networks for health monitoring [26]	Use of ad hoc networks to supplement infrastructure-oriented wireless networks for health monitoring. As part of providing reliability with power conservation, power management protocols and sleep cycles for monitoring devices are developed.
Demand-based design of wireless networks for healthcare applications [54]	The use of demand-based design for 3G networks. The placement of base stations could satisfy both coverage and data capacity for healthcare applications.

6.2 Evolution of WHM

The existing and emerging work in wireless health monitoring has been focusing on deriving requirements of various scenarios, describing visions, development of prototypes and wearable sensors, monitoring for preventive care and geriatric population and networking support for wireless health monitoring. This forms the first generation of wireless health monitoring system (WHMS), as shown in Figure 6.1(a). Thus, the first generation of WHMS provided wireless coverage and patient mobility and involved several prototypes and proof-of-concepts. The first generation of wireless health monitoring system involved monitoring devices ob-

taining and transmitting raw vital signs to a care center. The care center then decided if an alert/alarm was necessary to send to a certain healthcare professional.
Although there have been attempts to use off-the-shelf components in prototypes [2], specific and proprietary architectures would limit the interoperability among wireless health monitoring systems using a variety of wireless networks, thus affect the usability and wide-scale deployment of such systems (http://www.continuaalliance.org). As the monitoring environment evolves, such systems may not be able to adapt well due to their design optimizations for a specific set of monitoring conditions. This can be addressed by incorporating monitoring enhancements in middleware and application layers [19, 20]. These include context-awareness, inter-operability using middleware features, multi-network access, and adaptiveness to monitoring conditions. Also, with changes in monitoring requirements, additional functionalities in devices and wireless networks, and to support patients with multiple chronic health conditions, the wireless health monitoring is evolving to the second generation as shown in Figure 6.1(b). The devices, networks, and protocols for 2nd generation are likely to involve a higher degree of intelligence, context-awareness and adaptation to the changing wireless monitoring environment. In the second generation, wireless health monitoring (WHM) devices process vital signs locally before making a decision on whether to just store, transmit, and/or add any alert messages. The devices can be programmed with patient specific thresholds for vital signs along with patient information to make such decisions. The second generation WHMS also offer greater mobility with use of one or more wireless networks, unlike the common use of last-hop wireless network for devices in the first generation WHMS. The 2nd generation WHMS also allow transmission of vital signs and/or alert messages to one of several healthcare professionals thus improving the reliability of wireless health monitoring. The decision to send information to a specific healthcare professional can be made based on (a) network reachability (b) network traffic and distance, and (c) the current load of the healthcare professional. In practice, normal vital signs will be transmitted to the "assigned" healthcare professional, while emergency signals could be transmitted to the first available healthcare professional.
As part of the 2nd and future generations, wireless health monitoring should address many interesting and exciting challenges including management of multiple chronic conditions; personalized and patient-centric monitoring; improving the reliability of monitoring with advances in sensors and wearable technologies, reduction of noise in measurement, and power conservation; use of groups/friends to share monitoring information for better compliance with health and medical advice; and specialized monitoring of interesting problems/conditions.

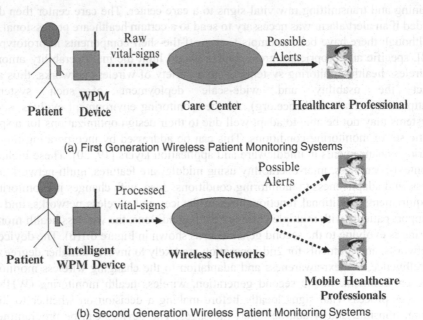

(a) First Generation Wireless Patient Monitoring Systems

(b) Second Generation Wireless Patient Monitoring Systems

Fig. 6.1 Generations of Wireless Health Monitoring Systems (WHMS)

6.3 A High-level Framework for WHM

In this section, a high-level framework for WHM is presented. The constraints, inputs and outputs, and desired performance of wireless health monitoring are shown in Figure 6.2. As the patients may be unlikely to intervene in the monitoring process, the framework should lead to adaptive and autonomous WHM systems to function well with evolving constraints. The framework components (Figure 6.3) adapt to monitoring environment by varying parameters. The middleware protocol adapts to the requirements of vital signs, number of patients, network traffic, and expected performance by varying message transmission priority, by switching to the transmission of only abnormal and urgent vital signs, and, choosing when to access wireless networks. The monitoring devices adapt to changing requirements such as reliability by managing power, and other requirements of vital signs by varying how often the vital signs are obtained, processed and transmitted. Wireless networks can adapt to changing reliability and interference by managing transmission at different power levels.

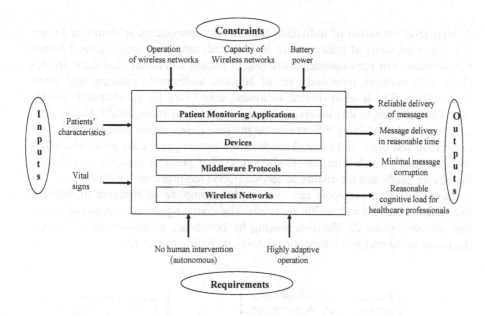

Fig. 6.2 The Constraints and Requirements for WHM framework

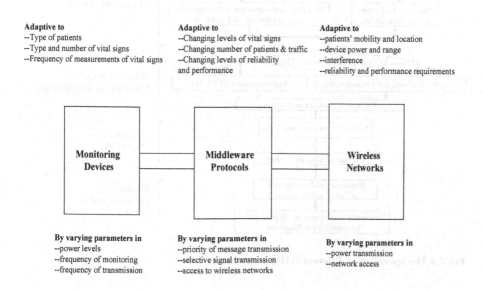

Fig. 6.3 The Adaptive Components of WHM Framework

A high-level operation of individual framework components is shown in Figure 6.4. The vital signs of patients must be obtained, amplified, and digitized before transmission. For personalized monitoring, a patient's nominal vital signs are defined with multiple thresholds, set of actions, undesirable patterns, and inter-relationships. The level of context-awareness could vary from a simple threshold-based comparison to that involving location, emotional states, health history, and activities, and to utilizing information on missing doses, recent labs, known handicaps, food and diets, and unusual conditions. Context-generation protocols, utilizing weighted probabilities and prediction, derive possible contexts of patient's healthcare needs and the quality of service (QoS) requirements for vital signs. The context-generation protocols can work with incomplete information in deriving the patient's context and healthcare needs. The context-generation protocols *assist* and do *not replace* the decision making by healthcare professionals, who make decisions using multiple informational items including the context.

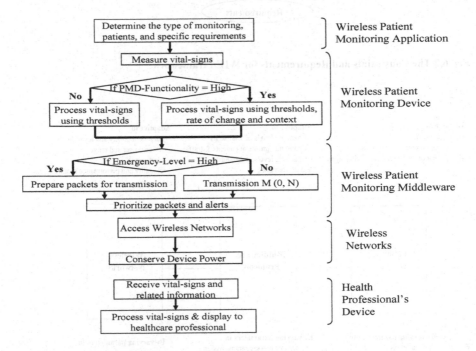

Fig. 6.4 The operation of different WHM components

As an example of vital signs processing, the patterns in ECG are processed as shown in Figure 6.5, which presents a simple example of using ECG components in alarm generation. In practice, more comprehensive algorithms will be utilized to approximate the goal of zero "false-negatives" or minimal false-positives. The framework is flexible enough to allow different alarm logics to be implemented with changes in the monitoring requirement. The framework could lead to data analysis and alarm logic for complex monitoring scenarios and patients' conditions.

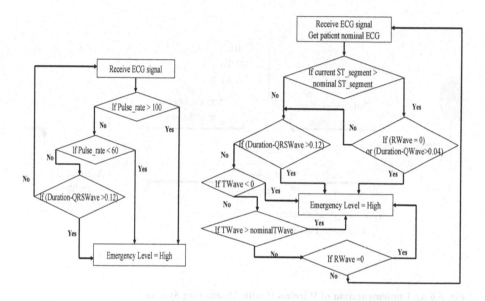

Fig. 6.5 Analysis of ECG signals for Alarm Generation

6.4 An Implementation

In this section, a possible implementation of WHM system using the framework is presented. The implementation consists of health monitoring devices, wireless network(s), devices for healthcare professionals, and storage of healthcare data and relevant medical information as shown in Figure 6.6. The processed vital signs, context and related information are transmitted through the underlying wireless network(s) to healthcare professionals. The personalized medical information and a set of actions, stored in a database, can be utilized for decision making by healthcare professionals. Wireless networks could also communicate with devices if needed, such as informing about the network conditions of traffic and/or failures. The wireless networks could also be informed by HP devices if an "alert" is being read by the HP or not. The capacity and speed of database storing the patient and medical information and the infrastructure between the database and HP devices may also affect the operation of WHM.

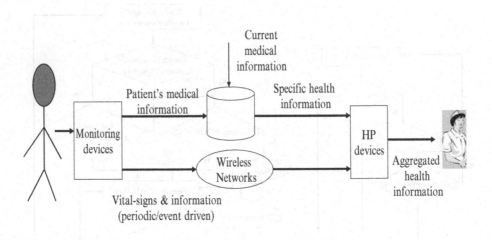

Fig. 6.6 An Implementation of Wireless Health Monitoring System

Wireless health monitoring involves measurement and digitization of vital signs, such as blood pressure (BP), Electrocardiogram (ECG), respiration rate, pulse, and oxygen saturation (SpO2) , transmission of packets over wireless networks, and delivery of medical information to healthcare professionals. The monitoring system should transmit both routine vital signs and alerting signals when vital signs cross one or more "individualized" thresholds. The vital signs are represented along with their nominal values in Figure 6.7. These vital signs are obtained, sampled, and digitized for transmission as network packets. The health monitoring device can be wearable or hand-held depending on the level of difficulty in use, portability, and the type of disability for the monitored patient. The devices should operate on their own and must send alarm signals when one or more problems arise. Once vital signs are obtained, they can be compared to different thresholds (values) to figure out if they are very low, low, normal, high or very high (Figure

6.7). Then one of several actions can be taken such as generating alerts/alarm if the vital sign is too low or too high.

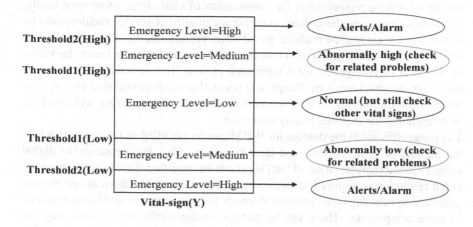

Fig. 6.7 Simple Threshold-based Processing of Vital Signs

The vital signs may have to be stored for processing later at a device or in a database. For personalized monitoring, patient's nominal vital signs are defined with multiple thresholds, set of actions, undesirable patterns, and inter-relationships.

6.4.1 Increasing Accuracy in Wireless Health Monitoring

One of the goals is to create wireless health monitoring with zero "false-negatives" where severity of patient's condition is not detected and minimal number of "false-positives" where the system overestimates the severity of patient's condition. The monitoring rules, individualized to the patient, are specified by a healthcare professional and could result in a more accurate generation of "alerts". Then, a threshold and pattern-based processing is performed to derive emergency level (Figure 6.8). For managing complexity, the rules for context-generation, modified as necessary by healthcare professionals, could be programmed to limit the possible contexts to cover the most likely problems. In addition to the current values of vital signs and patient-specific thresholds, the health monitoring system, to differentiate a multitude of situations, could also utilize physical location, physiological and emotional states, personal health history, and, current activities.

In addition, in case of the availability of sensors, such information could also be utilized with patient's history of medical information. The context-aware protocols will be utilized to derive the current context of patient's healthcare needs and the quality of service requirements for transmission of vital signs. More specifically, context-awareness can be utilized to derive the quality of service requirements by differentiating among the multiple possibilities represented by absolute values of vital signs and thresholds. Thus context-awareness can lead to a better derivation of the level of emergency for a monitored patient. The information on missing doses, recent labs, known handicaps, and unusual conditions will also be very useful in health monitoring. The information on the type of monitoring will also help in determining the required quality of service.

The parameters set in the devices for WHM can be modified as necessary to adjust the number of false positives and false negatives. Also, the frequency or digital samples based representation of vital signs can be modified if more accurate or detailed resolution is required in medical decision making. The devices can be programmed to run diagnostic routines to check for any errors or malfunction of one or more components. These can be done in backgrounds without requiring patient's involvement or causing inconvenience to the patient.

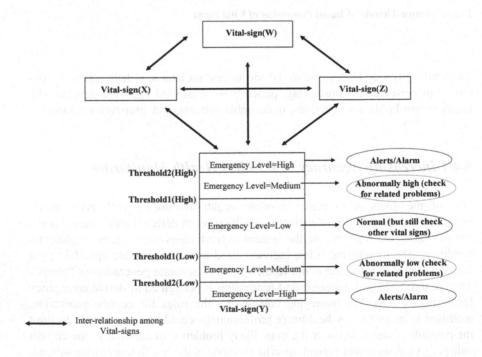

Fig. 6.8 Vital Signs and Multi-threshold based Processing

6.5 The Future of WHM

Wireless health monitoring will evolve to 2nd and future generations, where significantly higher reliability would be achieved. The patients with multiple chronic illnesses in multiple environments would be supported. The use of context-awareness would lead to more accurate and suitable medical decision making. It should be noted that there are many challenges that must be overcome before context-awareness becomes a common place. These include difficulty in adding functions and features in different components to make them context-aware. More work is also needed in making sure that the current and emerging regulatory environment, especially those pertaining to privacy and security, does not hinder deployment and usage of context-awareness in WHM.

The advances in non-invasive technologies to measure characteristics of blood and other fluids will allow continuous and reliable monitoring and will help patients to manage chronic conditions such as diabetes. This will reduce the incidence of uncontrolled blood sugar and hospitalization due to complications from chronic conditions.

The wireless health monitoring would become highly personalized and cost-effective due to flexibility, modifiability, re-configurability and re-usability of sensors, monitoring devices, and a range of wearable devices. A range of current and emerging wireless networks would be deployed in conjunction to improve the coverage, usability and reliability of wireless health monitoring. WHM systems would have the ability to monitor the quality of monitoring using multiple tools.

Questions:
1. List several requirements of wearable health monitoring systems. How are these different from portable health monitoring systems?
2. Discuss the problems of "all-in-one" health monitoring systems.
3. How would information from sensors/devices on one patient be differentiated from other patients?
4. Design and draw a "health wellness system" for healthy people who may be at risk, but have no history.
5. If we want to design more accurate monitoring systems with zero false-negatives and a few false-positives, what needs to be done?
6. What information may be needed in designing "personalized" health monitoring systems? Discuss.
7. Should other categories be added to improve the classification of the existing literature on wireless health monitoring and related areas? Why or why not?
8. What specific challenges may have to be dealt with in designing and implementing geriatric wireless health monitoring systems?

REFERENCES

[1]   Stefanov D, Bien Z, Bang W (2004) The smart house for older persons and persons with physical disabilities: structure, technology, arrangements, and perspectives. IEEE Trans Neural Syst Rehabil Eng 12(2):228–250, June

[2]   Jovanov E, Milenkovi A, Otto C, De Groen P, Johnson B, Warren S, Taibi G (2005) A WBAN system for ambulatory monitoring of physical activity and health status: applications and challenges. Proc. 27th Annu. Int. Conf. IEEE Eng. Med. Biol. Soc., 3810-3813

[3]   Lymberis A (2003) Smart wearable systems for personalised health management: current R&D and future challenges. Proc. 25th Annu. Int. Conf. IEEE Eng. Med. Biol. Soc., 3716-3719

[4]   Jovanov E, O'Donnel A, Morgan A, Priddy B, Hormigo R (2002) Prolonged telemetric monitoring of heart rate variability using wireless intelligent sensors and a mobile gateway. In Proc. Second Joint IEEE EMBS/BMES Conference, 1875–1876

[5]   Mendoza G, Tran B (2002) In-home wireless monitoring of physiological data for heart failure patients. Proc. 24th Annu. Int. Conf. IEEE Eng. Med. Biol. Soc. 1849-1850

[6]   Asada H, Shaltis P, Reisner A, Rhee S, Hutchinson R (2003) Mobile monitoring with wearable photoplethysmographic biosensors. IEEE Eng Med Biol Mag, 22(3):28–40, May–June

[7]   Liszka K, Mackin M, Lichter M, York D, Pillai D, Rosenbaum D (2004) Keeping a beat on the heart. IEEE Pervasive Computing Magazine, 42–49, Oct–Dec

[8]   Edström U, Skönevik J, Bäcklund T, Karlsson J (2005) A flexible measurement system for physiological signals in mobile health care. Proc. 27th Annu. Int. Conf. IEEE Eng. Med. Biol. Soc. 2161-2162

[9]   Lee R, Chen K, Hsiao C, Tseng C (2007) A mobile care system with alert mechanism. IEEE Trans. Inf. Technol. Biomed. 11(5):507-517, September

[10] Lin C, Chiu M, Hsiao C, Lee R, Tsai Y (2006) A wireless healthcare service system for elderly with dementia. IEEE Trans. Inf. Technol. Biomed, 10(2): 696-704, October

[11] Lin B, Chou N, Chong F, Chen S (2006) RTWPMS: a real-time wireless physiological monitoring system. IEEE Trans. Inf. Technol. Biomed, 10(4): 647-656, October

[12] Spenko M, Yu H, Dubowsky S (2006) Robotic personal aids for mobility and monitoring for the elderly. IEEE Trans. Neu. Syst. Rehab. Eng., 14(3):344-351, September

[13] Kang J, Yoo T, Kim H (2006) A wrist-worn integrated health monitoring instrument with a tele-reporting device for telemedicine and telecare. IEEE Trans. Instru. Measur. 55(5):1655-1661, Oct.

[14] Yu S, Cheng J (2005) A wireless physiological signal monitoring system with integrated bluetooth and WiFi technologies. Proc. 27th Annu. Int. Conf. IEEE Eng. Med. Biol. Soc. 2203-2206

[15] Otto C, Jovanov E, Milenkovic A (2006) A WBAN-based system for health monitoring at home. 3rd IEEE/EMBS Int. Summer School Medical Devices Biosensors, 20-23

[16] Kafeza E, Chiu D, Cheung S, Kafeza M (2004) Alerts in mobile healthcare applications: requirements and pilot study. IEEE Trans. Inf. Technol. Biomed, 8(2):173-181, June

[17] Varshney U (2006) Patient monitoring using infrastructure-oriented wireless LANs. Int. J. on Electronic Healthcare, 2(2):149-163

[18] Varshney U (2006) Managing wireless health monitoring for patients with disabilities. IEEE IT Professional, 8(6):12-16, Nov.-Dec.

[19] Hung K, Zhang Y-T (2003) Implementation of a WAP-based telemedicine system for patient monitoring. IEEE Trans. Inf. Technol. Biomed, 7(2):101-107, June

[20] Hu F, Wang Y, Wu H (2006) Mobile telemedicine sensor networks with low-energy data query and network lifetime considerations", IEEE Trans. Mob. Comp., 5(4):404-417, April

[21] Anliker U, Ward J, Luckowicz P, et al (2004) AMON: A wearable multiparameter medical monitoring and alert system. IEEE Trans on IT in Biomedicine 8(4):415–427, Dec.

[22] Modarreszadeh S (1997) Wireless, 32-channel, EEG and epilepsy monitoring system. In Proc. 19th Annual IEEE International Conference on Engineering in Medicine and Biology, 1157-1160

[23] Gieras I (2003) The proliferation of patient-worn wireless telemetry technologies within the U.S. healthcare environment. In Proc. 4th International IEEE EMBS Special Topic Conference on Information Technology Applications in Biomedicine, 295-298

[24] Khoor S, Nieberl K, Fugedi K, Kail E (2001) Telemedicine ECG-telemetry with Bluetooth technology. In Proc. Computers in Cardiology, 585-588

[25] Kyu J, Asada H (2002) Wireless, battery-less stethoscope for wearable health monitoring. In Proc. the IEEE 28th Annual Northeast Bioengineering Conference, 187-188

[26] Varshney U, Sneha S (2006) Patient monitoring using ad hoc wireless networks: reliability and power management. IEEE Communications Magazine, 44(4): 49-55, April

[27] Suzuki T, Doi M (2001) LifeMinder: an evidence-based wearable healthcare assistant. In Proc. ACM CHI Conference, March-April

[28] Istepanian R, Petrosian A (2000) Optimal zonal wavelet-based ECG data compression for a mobile telecardiology system. IEEE Trans on IT in Biomedicine 4(3):200-211, Sept

[29] Pavlopoulos S, Kyriacou E, Berler A, Dembeyiotis S, Koutsouris D (1998) Novel emergency telemedicine system based on wireless communication technology-AMBULANCE. IEEE Transactions on Information Technology in Biomedicine, 2(4):261-267, Dec.

[30] Rasid M, Woodward B (2005) Bluetooth telemedicine processor for multichannel biomedical signal transmission via mobile cellular networks. IEEE Transactions on Information Technology in Biomedicine, 9(1): 35-43, March

[31] Jianchu Y, Schmitz R, Warren S (2005) A wearable point-of-care system for home use that incorporates plug-and-play and wireless standards. IEEE Transactions on Information Technology in Biomedicine, 9(3): 363-371, Sept.

[32] Fort A, Ryckaert J, Desset C, Doncker P, Wambacq P, Van Biesen L (2006) Ultrawideband channel model for communication around the human body. IEEE Journal on Selected Areas in Communications, 24(4):927-933, April

[33] Bottazzi D, Corradi A, Montanari R (2006) Context-aware middleware solutions for anytime and anywhere emergency assistance to elderly people. IEEE Communications Magazine, 44(4):82-90, April

[34] Korhonen I, Parkka J, Gils M (2003) Health monitoring in the home of the future. IEEE Eng Med Biol Mag, 66–73, May–June

[35] Paradiso R, Loriga G, Taccini N (2005) A wearable health care system based on knitted integrated sensors. IEEE Transactions on IT in Biomedicine 9(3):337-344, Sept.

[36] Bhargava A, Zoltowski M (2003) Sensors and wireless communication for medical care. In Proc. 14th International Workshop on Database and Expert Systems Applications, 956-960

[37] Parkka J, Frumento E, Rentto K, Suihkonen R, Wersch O., Saranummi N (2002) Scenarios for health management in Future Home. Proceedings of the Second Joint 24th Annual Conference and the Annual Fall Meeting of the Biomedical Engineering Society-EMBS/BMES Conference, 1904–1905

[38] Warren S, Yao J, Schmitz R, Nagl L (2003) Wearable telemonitoring systems designed with interoperability in mind. Proceedings of the 25th Annual International Conference of the IEEE Engineering in Medicine and Biology Society, 3736-3739

[39] Konstantas D, Herzog R (2003) Continuous monitoring of vital constants for mobile users: the MobiHealth approach. Proceedings of the 25th Annual International Conference of the IEEE Engineering in Medicine and Biology Society, 3728–3731

[40] Isais R, Nguyen K, Perez G, Rubio R, Nazeran H (2003) A low-cost microcontroller-based wireless ECG-blood pressure telemonitor for home care. Proceedings of the 25th Annual International Conference of the IEEE Engineering in Medicine and Biology Society, 3157-3160

[41]   Rahman F, Kumar A, Nagendra G (2003) Network approach for physiological parameters measurement. Proceedings of the 20th IEEE Instrumentation and Measurement Technology Conference, 901-905

[42]   Gouaux F, Simon-Chautemps L, Adami S, Arzi M, Assanelli D, Fayn J, Forlini M, Malossi C, Martinez A, Placide J, Ziliani G, Rubel P (2003) Smart devices for the early detection and interpretation of cardiological syndromes. 4th International IEEE EMBS Special Topic Conference on Information Technology Applications in Biomedicine, 291-294

[43]   Susan L. Mabry, Troy Schneringer, Timothy Etters, and Naomi Edwards (2003) Intelligent agents for patient monitoring and diagnostics. Proceedings of the 2003 ACM symposium on Applied computing, pp. 257 – 262

[44]   Venugopal M, Feuvrel K, Mongin D, Bambot S, Faupel M, Panangadan A, Talukder A, Pidva R (2008) Clinical evaluation of a novel interstitial fluid sensor system for remote continuous alcohol monitoring. IEEE Sensors Journal, 8(1):71-80, January

[45]   Falck T, Baldus H, Espina J, Klabunde K (2006) Plug 'n play simplicity for wireless medical body sensors. Proceedings of First International Conference on Pervasive Computing Technologies for Healthcare (IEEE)

[46]   Carlos G. Bilich (2006) Bio-medical sensing using ultra wideband communications and radar technology: a feasibility study. Proceedings of First International Conference on Pervasive Computing Technologies for Healthcare (IEEE)

[47]   Maitland J, Sherwood S, Barkhuus L, Anderson I, Hall M, Brown B, Chalmers M, Muller H (2006) Increasing the awareness of daily activity levels with pervasive computing. Proceedings of First International Conference on Pervasive Computing Technologies for Healthcare (IEEE)

[48]   Oliver N, Kreger-Stickles L (2006) Enhancing exercise performance through real-time physiological monitoring and music: a user study. Proceedings of First International Conference on Pervasive Computing Technologies for Healthcare (IEEE)

[49]   Tsai C, Lee G, Raab F, Norman G, Sohn T, Griswold W, Patrick K (2006) Usability and feasibility of PMEB: a mobile phone application for monitoring real time caloric balance, Proceedings of First International Conference on Pervasive Computing Technologies for Healthcare (IEEE)

[50]   Amft O, Troster G (2006) Methods for detection and classification of normal swallowing from muscle activation and sound. Proceedings of First International Conference on Pervasive Computing Technologies for Healthcare (IEEE)

[51]   Parkka J, Ermes M, Korpipaa P, Mantyjarvi J, Peltola J, Korhonen I (2006) Activity classification using realistic data from wearable sensors. IEEE Trans. Inf. Technol. Biomed. 10(1): 119-128, Jan.

[52]   Karantonis D, Narayanan M, Mathie M, Lovell N, Celler B (2006) Implementation of a real-time human movement classifier using a triaxial accelerometer for ambulatory monitoring. IEEE Trans. Inf. Technol. Biomed. 10(1): 156-167, Jan.

[53]   Boger J, Hoey J, Poupart P, Boutilier C, Fernie G, Mihailidis A (2006) A planning system based on markov decision processes to guide people with dementia through activities of daily living. IEEE Trans. Inf. Technol. Biomed. 10(2): 323-333, April.

[54]   Pongthaipat N, Kabara J (2006) Designing wireless networks to support data rate requirements of healthcare systems. Proceedings of First International Conference on Pervasive Computing Technologies for Healthcare (IEEE)

[55]   S. Intille (2004) A new research challenge: persuasive technology to motivate healthy aging. IEEE Trans. Inf. Technol. Biomed. 8(3): 235-237, Sept.

[56]   Virone G, Alwan M, Dalal S, Kell S, Turner B, Stankovic J, Felder, R (2008) Behavioral patterns of older adults in assisted living. IEEE Trans. Inf. Technol. Biomed. 12(3): 387-398, May.

Chapter 7 Medical Decision Making

Abstract In wireless health monitoring, healthcare professionals will make decisions based on knowledge derived from multiple sets of informational items such as patient's medical history, current vital signs, medical knowledge, and specific patient conditions. In this chapter, we discuss medical decision making process by focusing on devices of healthcare professionals, requirements and functions of healthcare professionals, what to do when something goes wrong, and, how to manage cognitive load. We also present a monitoring system with four components to monitor generation, transmission, processing and impacts of various alerts. Finally, how the medical decisions may be made in the future is presented.

7.1 Introduction

The purpose of wireless health monitoring is to minimize care when not necessary, deliver care to minimize near-future episodes of serious nature, and provide medical help as quickly as possible when an emergency has occurred. This preventive and efficient delivery of healthcare services may be different from "reactive" and episodic model of diagnosis and treatment. Wireless health monitoring (WHM) could support mobility of "monitored" patients and also of healthcare professionals, who can then be more efficiently utilized to perform other tasks and alerted only when changes occur in patients' conditions. Wireless health monitoring will also allow more un-obtrusive monitoring of a patient's chronic diseases, and could obtain more realistic vital signs and biomedical parameters as patients conduct daily activities without being confined to beds or certain locations. Several health parameters, including weight, sleep patterns and activities, can be autonomously measured by embedding sensors in bed, toilet, bathtub, and kitchen appliances. These will also improve decision making by healthcare professionals and eventually a better level of health and quality of life for patients. Most of the work in wireless health monitoring involves dealing with how to obtain vital signs and transmit to a healthcare professional for decision making. What healthcare professionals must do and how their devices can assist them in performing their medical decision making have not been sufficiently addressed. Therefore, we discuss the requirements and functions of healthcare professionals in this chapter.

In wireless health monitoring, healthcare professionals will make decisions based on knowledge derived from multiple sets of informational items such as patient's medical history, current vital signs, medical knowledge, and specific patient conditions. Figure 7.1 shows how medical information can be represented for individual patients to achieve a high degree of personalization. The vital signs are defined with multiple thresholds, sets of actions, undesirable patterns, and inter-relationship between multiple vital signs. The representation of medical informa-

U. Varshney, *Pervasive Healthcare Computing: EMR/EHR, Wireless and Health Monitoring*,   147
DOI: 10.1007/978-1-4419-0215-3_7,
© Springer Science + Business Media, LLC 2009

tion will be helpful for designing a comprehensive health monitoring system by utilizing both stored and live information. This along with the patient's current context (surroundings, patient's current activity, and emotional/physical states) will lead to a more suitable action by healthcare professionals. Comprehensive wireless health monitoring system should be actively context-aware, which will also aid in a better decision making by healthcare professionals on patient's current conditions and healthcare needs. In health monitoring, users can be patients whose primary task is being monitored for one or more health conditions and receive necessary medical attention, or healthcare professionals, whose primary task is to receive current and accurate information on monitored patients and perform decision making on patients' conditions and required care.

The context-generation protocols can be designed to assist and not replace the medical decision making by healthcare professionals, who make decisions using multiple informational items including the context. The protocols can be stored and processed in the health monitoring devices that a patient can carry or wear as a part of smart clothing. The context-generation protocols can be modified to work with incomplete and/or missing information in deriving the patient's context and healthcare needs.

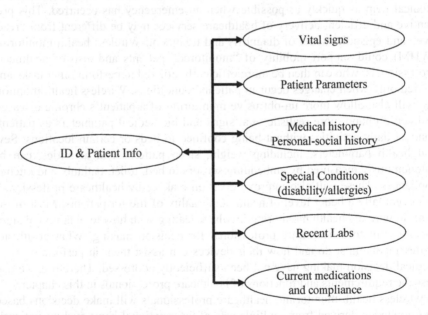

Fig. 7.1 Representation of Patient Information

7.2 Requirements and Functions of Healthcare Professionals

In this section, various requirements for healthcare professionals are identified and discussed (Figure 7.2). One major point that should be added here is that acceptance of mobile decision making by healthcare professionals is critical to effective decision making. The training of healthcare professionals in medical and allied health schools in mobile decision making could be very beneficial in such acceptance.

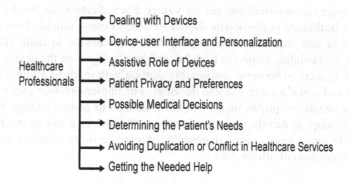

Healthcare Professionals
- Dealing with Devices
- Device-user Interface and Personalization
- Assistive Role of Devices
- Patient Privacy and Preferences
- Possible Medical Decisions
- Determining the Patient's Needs
- Avoiding Duplication or Conflict in Healthcare Services
- Getting the Needed Help

Fig. 7.2 Requirements of Healthcare Professionals

7.2.1 Dealing with Devices

The healthcare professionals should have the training and experience in dealing with a range of display sizes, devices' inputs and outputs, and patients. In pervasive healthcare environment, healthcare professionals may be provided with one or more devices capable of receiving and displaying patient's information, current vital signs, and stored medical information. The devices are likely to be small hand-held devices, but in some cases, healthcare professionals may be able to display information on larger screens or displays in certain areas, such as those in a hospital or clinic [3]. These screens may be context-aware and could display necessary information based on the presence of certain healthcare professionals in their vicinity. But some precaution must be taken to avoid displaying patient information when other people, not directly involved in the care of patient, are present.

However, the limitation of screen size may not be completely overcome as healthcare professionals may have to deal with smaller screens of hand-held devices in places without the large displays, such as outside a building or on the road.

7.2.2 Device-user Interface and Personalization

The healthcare professionals will receive vital signs, patient parameters, and alerts. This should be provided to them in a format/form suitable for decision making, also known as medically meaningful way. The user interface is important here as it should allow quick reading of different parameters. It may be desirable to display the most important or minimal information first, followed by more detailed information as needed or requested by healthcare professionals. The patient's parameters that are out of range can also be color coded, such as green for normal, orange for abnormal and red for values that indicate some level of emergency. The healthcare professionals should be able to move quickly between different screens and should be able to personalize the device to their individual working style, including setting of how "alerts" be displayed on the device screen. This will help them to be more comfortable dealing with medical information and vital signs and make a more suitable decision. For implementation purposes, the devices for healthcare professionals can be initialized to certain setting, then the devices can adapt to healthcare professionals or the interface can be modified as necessary. In many cases, visual representation may be more effective than text-based representation of information.

7.2.3 Assistive Role of Devices

The healthcare professional should be able to make decisions in the environment, where technologies are designed to assist and not replace the decision making of healthcare professionals. This could involve ignoring potential suggestions from devices. This could include overwriting an "alert" if necessary, or if the device suggests several options in a decreasing probability, the healthcare professional should be able to consider all the options including the one with a lower probability and not be completely influenced by automated processing of devices. In some case, when working with context-aware systems, sometimes the device interface may get updated, making the HP feels that she is loosing control as observed by [4]. It may be possible that another alert may arrive for a different patient, while decision making for the previous one is not completed. The healthcare professional should have the training to address these challenges that may be created by supportive technology in trying to assist the healthcare professional.

7.2.4 Patient Privacy and Preferences

The healthcare professional should be able to make the necessary and informed medical decision for the patient, while providing the privacy and respecting the patient's preferences, even if unreasonable.

The privacy challenge may become more difficult due to the mobility of the healthcare professional and potential for people nearby that are not directly related to patient's healthcare services. But to satisfy both the patient's need for privacy and also to regulatory frameworks such as HIPAA, the healthcare professional would have to be careful not to disclose sensitive information to someone not directly related to patient's healthcare.

In some cases, patients may have stated preference for what medical care should be provided in certain cases such as DNR: do not resuscitate. The decision making should support such "personalized" healthcare. In practice, the final decision may have to satisfy patient's preference, even though it may not be the best decision from the point of view of patient' current health needs.

7.2.5 Possible Medical Decisions

The healthcare professional may face one of the following situations:

- The patient's current condition is normal and no medical help is necessary. In this case, a simple message to the patient and/or designated family members could be sent if possible.
- The patient's current condition is normal, but a reminder about a "missed" medication is necessary. In such case, a message can be sent to the patient or caregiver using the desired form of communications.
- The patient's current condition is not normal, but is not serious enough for hospitalization. A simple phone call or text-message to the legal guardian should be enough. In some countries, the patient must also be notified while in some countries there are laws against such notification.
- The patient's condition is serious and needs hospitalization. The information on patients is communicated to the hospital for proactive management of facilities. The designated family members and/or caregiver should ne notified.
- The current situation is not an emergency, but more information is necessary to make a suitable decision. In this case, some attempts could be made to collect the missing/needed information and then suitable decision could be made.

7.2.6 Determining the Patient's Needs

Once the patient's current information is received and displayed on the healthcare professional's device, the healthcare professional must determine the patient's needs. In addition to vital signs, possible "alert" message from patient monitoring device, and patient's medical history (EMR), the healthcare professional may also have access to context information. In some cases, there may be additional information on sleep pattern and medication compliance. The healthcare professional may also acquire more information about the patient such as stored information, information from online or m-pharmacy, patient's preferences, and more details on context. One of the major challenges is to figure out the right action out of several choices for different scenarios. The healthcare professional has to figure out what is the problem, what is the diagnosis, what is the treatment, who to contact, and where to deliver what services. The problem could be figured out using the information and vital signs available. For diagnosis, there are several possibilities. For chronic conditions, some diagnosis may already have been made and healthcare professional may only have to figure out one of several actions for the current condition, such as sending medical help to patient's home. When a prior diagnosis is not available, medical decision making may become more complex and one of the several following actions may have to be taken:

- In some cases, delay the final decision making before more information/additional vital signs arrive or being able to work with a set of preliminary diagnoses before reaching to a final one
- Able to work with other HP in quickly receiving/providing some help in decision making

It is very important for the healthcare professional to be able to make "informed" decisions under incomplete and/or incorrect information. In most cases, figuring out the level and type of emergency is more important than the exact diagnosis, which can be done later by a physician or another qualified healthcare professional.

7.2.7 Avoiding Conflict in Healthcare Services

Normally, a certain number of patients under monitoring will be assigned to a healthcare professional, who will receive their information on a periodic or as needed basis for decision making. But in case the "designated" healthcare professional can not be reached by the underlying wireless networks or the level of emergency is high, such designation may not be followed. In this case, the information may reach to any one or even multiple healthcare professionals. This could lead to several undesirable scenarios including duplication of services if two or more healthcare professionals come up with the same set of medical decisions or conflicts in healthcare delivery if the decision making by two or more healthcare professionals happened to be quite different. The system could be programmed to check with the next-level healthcare professional if for some reason, duplicated or conflicted decisions are made.

To avoid such cases, one of several things can be done. These include (a) allowing only one HP to receive the information and if the HP does not acknowledge in a certain time then the next HP is contacted, (b) allowing more than one HP to receive the information but accept the first completed decision. Both of these have their advantages and disadvantages. The first option may take more time, but conflicts or duplication will not arise. In the second option, it will be faster to make a decision and as soon as decision by one healthcare professional is completed, the monitoring system should immediately update the screens of other healthcare professionals who are still in the decision making process.

7.2.8 Working on Getting the Needed Help

Once a medical decision has been made, which also addresses patient's preferences and privacy requirements, the next step is to get the necessary medical help to the patient in his/her current location. The patient's current location is likely to affect how the necessary action is implemented. For example, if the patient's current location is his/her home, and the healthcare professional evaluates that the level of emergency is high, then the set of actions include

- Informing the legal guardian of the patient
- Sending an ambulance to the patient's current location
- Possibly communicating with the patient and giving some instructions on what he/she could do
- Informing the hospital about the current conditions of the patient and expected arrival of patient to that facility

If the patient's current location is a nursing home, then the healthcare professional could call an emergency number to get ambulance while also reaching to the patient to provide any needed care. The actions can be similarly implemented for other scenarios involving patients living at assisted living, hospital or generally mobile within an area or city. The decision to inform the legal guardian of a patient or the patient herself could also be influenced by the regulatory framework as some countries allow the patient to be notified if something is not normal in the monitored signs, while others have rules against such notification.

7.3 The Role of Healthcare Professionals' Devices

The devices will play a major, yet supportive role, in decision making by healthcare professionals. The following is a list of requirements and useful functions of these devices (Figure 7.3). Please note that some of these are required, some useful functions are possible today and some will become possible in the near future. Additionally, some functions will be nice to have in the future to improve the quality of wireless health monitoring.

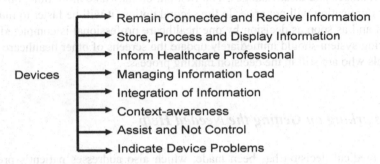

Devices

- Remain Connected and Receive Information
- Store, Process and Display Information
- Inform Healthcare Professional
- Managing Information Load
- Integration of Information
- Context-awareness
- Assist and Not Control
- Indicate Device Problems

Fig. 7.3 Requirements and Functions of HP Devices

7.3.1 Remain Connected and Reliably Receive Information

One of the major functions of healthcare professionals' devices is maintain their network connectivity even when the healthcare professionals are mobile and/or network is experiencing one of several problems. The ability to access more than one network in a location will help in remain connected, but devices may have to make such decision to switch to another network. The devices must also receive information (packets) in a reliable fashion and filter away any duplicate information.

7.3.2 Store, Process and Display Information

The devices should be able to store, process and display a range of patient and medical information in a style suited to their healthcare professionals. This will help in making suitable medical decision by the healthcare professional. In some cases, the devices could proactively download information which may assist in decision making.

7.3.3 Inform HP about the Current Situation

The wireless health monitoring environment is very dynamic where information about patients, networks, devices and other people could change quickly. The devices should be able to prioritize information, especially if context can be utilized. The devices should be able to communicate this information to HP as quickly as possible in the best possible way. Based on the response from the healthcare professional, the devices should also be able to "react" to the changing environment.

7.3.4 Manage Loads for HP

One of the ways where a device can assist in decision making is to manage load for its healthcare professional. In some cases, it may keep track of how many alerts have been processed or transmitted to a HP and how long it has taken, then decide who to sent the "alert" in case there is some choice. In general, some pre-processing may be done to assist the HP in making a suitable decision.

7.3.5 Information Integration

The HP device will have to integrate information from several places and this could include vital signs, EMR, medical information, and any recent warnings. This should be done without sacrificing the quality of information. Therefore, the device should continuously try to get as accurate and current information as possible to improve the decision making for healthcare professionals. The speed of downloading information from potentially multiple places may affect the service quality to the patient. More work is needed in devising how much information can be downloaded, filtered, stored and processed by HP devices.

7.3.6 Role of Context-awareness

The HP devices may be context-aware or be part of context-aware wireless health monitoring system. As part of this, the devices could monitor the monitoring load and cognitive load of healthcare professional. If the decision is taking longer, these can try to communicate with HP if some more information is needed or indicate that some new information may have become available. If context is partial or incorrect, then the devices should know how to deal with it including waiting to get more information or not considering it at all for the time being.

7.3.7 Assist and not Control the Decision Making

The devices should help in medical decision making-based on personalized settings of the healthcare professional. The devices should also help when there is some difficulty in medical decision making due to incomplete information, and/or lack of training/knowledge of HP. The devices should not replace the human decision making.

7.3.8 Indicate Problems to HP

The device should be able to indicate any problems in battery, network coverage, failures, processing, delays, and, incorrect integration/display to the healthcare professional to help in decision making. This is in addition to periodic maintenance, repair and replacements and use of diagnostic programs to check for errors and problems in the device in advance.

7.4 An Example of Medical Decision Making

The devices used by healthcare professionals (HPs), an important component in the reliability of health monitoring, will receive patient information, vital signs, and context information from patient monitoring devices, perform processing, and inform or alert healthcare professionals. The architecture and components of healthcare professional's device are shown in Figure 7.4. To implement these functions, the devices for HP will perform the following operations:
1. Get vital signs from patient monitoring devices via wireless network(s)
2. Filter duplicate packets using sequence number and patient identification number
3. Download patient medical information from EMR database
4. Integrate and display information and alerts for healthcare professional
5. Inform devices of other healthcare professionals to avoid duplicate/conflicting set of actions.

A simple flow chart implementing some of the functions is presented in Figure 7.5. To decide if this healthcare professional should receive monitored information, the patient-ID must be matched with the IDs of patients allocated to the healthcare professional (Patient_ID = HP[I]). However, in cases of emergency level being high, such checks are not performed and the healthcare professional will perform decision making as necessary.

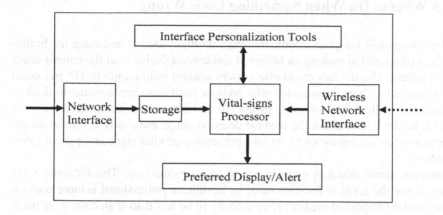

Fig. 7.4 Architecture of the Healthcare Professional's Device

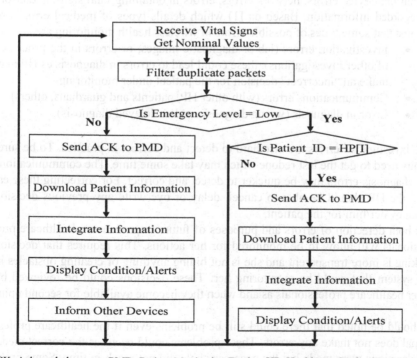

ACK: Acknowledgement, PMD: Patient Monitoring Device, HP: Healthcare Professional

Fig. 7.5 Some Functions of HP Device

7.5 What to Do When Something Goes Wrong

The devices will integrate information from multiple sources and assist the health-care professional in making an informed and correct decision on the current needs of a patient. The devices could also present context information to HP and could also support a short consultation with another healthcare professional to double-check the medical decision made by the HP. In addition, device could also ask the HP if he/she is sure about the medical decision made, especially if the device detects obvious discrepancies by its own processing of vital signs and patient information.

However, some mistakes could occur in certain situations. The fortunate thing here is that the medical decision made by healthcare professional is more preliminary and the impact of medical error is likely to be less than if an error were made in the final diagnosis. For practice, the goal of WHM is to have zero false negatives, where the HP incorrectly detects a lower or no level of emergency, but a few false-positives, where the HP incorrectly detects a higher level of emergency, could be tolerated. The number of such false positives should be minimized to reduce waste of healthcare resources.

The errors or incorrect decisions could occur due to problems in the quality of information, device errors, network errors, errors in obtaining vital signs, and errors in recorded information. Based on [1] which details types of medical errors, we suggest that some types of possible errors in wireless health monitoring are:

- Investigation errors (lab or diagnostic images, or errors in the processes of other investigations): these could lead to errors in diagnosis as HP may make an "incorrect" decision for the patient under monitoring
- Communications errors (with other HP, patients and guardians, others)
- Error in diagnosis (wrong diagnosis and/or delayed diagnosis)

The investigative errors are also hard to detect and correct in practice. To be sure, it may need to get the test redone which may take some time. The communications and diagnosis errors may be quicker to detect and correct. For correcting these errors, the HP should be able to cancel, delay or overwrite any previous decision made by her/him for the patient.

For both detection of errors and purposes of future improvement, healthcare professionals will allow to be monitored for her actions. This requires that decision making is more transparent and she is not hiding anything or creating obstacles in the system that could be monitoring her. These decisions could be reviewed by other healthcare professionals as and when they become available for second opinion.

It should be noted that there could still be problems even if the healthcare professional does not make any errors. These problems could occur as the correct medical decisions were made but the necessary help did not reach in time. Some problems could also occur due to duplication in healthcare services, which could be minimized by the HP by keeping track of what services have been delivered and what has been ordered by her. Another factor which can contribute to medical errors is the potential cognitive load of healthcare professionals involved in WHM.

7.6 Cognitive Load

Due to the number of patients that are under monitoring, the number of messages that are generated, and the number of actions that must be taken, healthcare professionals could feel very overwhelm during some part of the health monitoring. This may be exacerbated by the small screens and other limitations of devices used in decision making. Although healthcare professionals may have different levels of processing abilities needed in medical decision making, more work is needed in evaluating how the monitoring load will affect the decision making ability in terms of errors. One of the factors is cognitive load, which refers to load on working memory, usually short-term memory and may also relate to the number of units of information that can be retained in short term memory before information loss occurs [2]. Thus, excessive cognitive load may negatively affect the quality of medical decision making in terms of number of errors.

Although, there are possibly large variation in the cognitive resources (working memory and reasoning skills), some factors could affect the cognitive load of healthcare professionals perfuming medical decision making. These could include factors such as the tendency to multitask, lack of sleep and rest, and mental tiredness in general. Certainly, these could be included in the training and work load of healthcare professionals to address cognitive load. It is possible that the need to translate information by a healthcare professional, whose first language is not English or the language used in decision making, contributes to an increased cognitive load.

Severe cognitive load could lead to errors and fundamental attributional errors [2]. The fundamental attributional errors involve blaming an action of a person on his/her personality and not on the social and environmental forces. These could have major implications on health monitoring as healthcare professionals may attribute some alerts to the patient's personality and not on the current difficult situation the patient may be in. Certainly, more work is needed in identifying the impact of cognitive load on types of errors and the ways for a monitoring system to carefully watch those errors.

7.6.1 Managing Cognitive Load

One of the important factors in the success of wireless health monitoring is the ability to keep the cognitive load of healthcare professionals to a reasonable level.

The ability to work with mobile devices and the ability to personalize the devices to suit their working style may help reduce the cognitive load.

The number of messages that must be received and processed by healthcare professionals could be used as a measure of cognitive load. Such load can vary widely based on the frequency of monitoring, number of patients that must be monitored, number of messages per monitored event, and the number of healthcare professionals involved. There are many ways to manage the cognitive load including increasing the number of healthcare professionals, reducing the frequency of monitoring, and filtering or combining packets. Also, many other improvements could be added such as the use of un-even load to match individual abilities of healthcare professionals, use of context-awareness of which healthcare professional is currently busy in messages, and adapting of parameters to the current load of healthcare professionals. The number of messages can also be reduced by message filtering at healthcare professional's device using sequence number and patient id. This additional information in a packet will lead to an increased overhead at the network due to larger sized packets and also any incorrect filtering of packets could lead to problems for a certain patient.

7.6.2 Future Work in Cognitive Load

Certainly much more work needs to be done in creating best set of work and environmental conditions for HPs to generate best medical decisions for patients under monitoring. This could include design of devices that can present various information items to the most natural way to individual healthcare professional and adapt to his/her style of performing various mental tasks involved in medical decision making. This would become difficult to achieve if there are cyclic variations in how a healthcare professional performs certain tasks. Some of the decisions should also be stored to be shown to the healthcare professional for further training and possible improvement in decision making abilities. There has been some evidence that the way information is presented, symbolic vs textual, may influence the cognitive load. It is shown that symbolic presentation of information may be more efficient from the cognitive point and could lead to faster response and fewer errors in acute care [5].

7.7 Alert Monitoring and Management System

To address and manage the alerts in health monitoring, an alert management system can be designed as shown in Figure 7.6. The AMS has four components: Monitoring of Alert Generation, Monitoring of Alert Transmission, Monitoring of Alert Processing, and Monitoring of Updates. The AMS can be added on top of any health monitoring system to evaluate how well the alerts are managed in the monitoring system at several different places. The AMS does generate some overhead and is flexible enough to run continuously or intermittently based on the desired level of additional overhead to health monitoring system. It is also possible to just employ one of AMS components, such as Monitoring of Alert Processing to evaluate how well the healthcare professionals are making medical decisions.

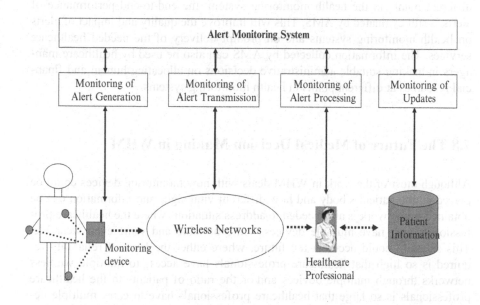

Fig. 7.6 Alert Monitoring System to Evaluate the Effectiveness of Alerts in Health Monitoring

The basic function of AMS is as follows. Each generated alert is assigned a sequence number. This will allow both filtering of duplicated messages as well as analysis of the effectiveness of alert generation, transmission and processing. The alert generation at monitoring devices will be analyzed later to see how many false positive and false negative alerts have been generated and what parameters can be adjusted to increase the effectiveness, or control the frequency, of future alert generation. Similarly, the transmission of alerts over wireless networks can be analyzed to evaluate the effectiveness of networks in delivering the alerts to healthcare professionals. This could allow for fine tuning of various parameters, including the use of higher priority and higher persistency level in network protocols. Similarly, how well the alerts are processed by healthcare professionals can be analyzed and one or more guidelines on improving the quality of decision making can be generated and communicated to HPs. The AMS will allow monitoring of the quality of decision making and may be able to evaluate if there are mistakes and what can be done. It can also be used to check if mistakes in alert processing may be related to the cognitive load of HPs or any behavioral issues such as outright ignoring of alerts in some cases. The AMS also allows for monitoring of various updates and can process these to detect any anomalous information, entered during or after the processing of an alert.

Although the four different components of AMS can be used to monitor alerts at different points in the health monitoring system, the end-to-end performance of alerts is still evaluated by AMS. This will improve the quality and impact of alerts on health monitoring systems and on prompt delivery of the needed healthcare services. The information collected by AMS can also be used by healthcare managers in making suitable administrative decisions on allocating human and financial resources at different points in health monitoring systems.

7.8 The Future of Medical Decision Making in WHM

Although most of the work in WHM deals with how monitoring devices could be placed on the patient's body and how different vital signs and information can be obtained, some work is also needed to address situations where the healthcare professionals may have multiple devices, some portable and some even wearable. This situation could occur in the future, where either the level of reliability required is so high that healthcare professionals have access to multiple wireless networks through multiple devices and/or the ratio of patients to the healthcare professionals is so large that healthcare professionals have to carry multiple devices for medical decision making. In general, multiple devices will allow a higher reliability of WHM as the network could reach at least one of those devices even when one or more of the devices have problems or are already involved in ongoing alerts. Then context could be used to decide which device to be used to transmit the vital signs and alert. To support this scenario, some communications between these multiple devices may be required, thus there would be a need to create a network among these devices, such as a personal area network or a body area network. More work may be needed to avoid any conflicts or deadlocks, caused due to large amount of information and limited storage resources on these devices. How the context could be generated, processed, transmitted and utilized in decision making is also an important area of research. Certainly more work is needed in evaluating the working conditions and stress levels of healthcare professionals in wireless health monitoring and pervasive health environments. What factors will affect the medical decision making and in what proportion, should also be evaluated.

Questions
1. Discuss two roles of healthcare professional's devices in medical decision making.
2. What do healthcare professionals need to do for accurate or suitable medical decision making?
3. What needs to be done when something goes wrong in decision making?
4. What is cognitive load and how it affects the quality of medical decision making?
5. Explore more details on cognitive load and ways to reduce it including visual representation of information and display of information related to the current episode only.
6. Derive the protocol steps that will be used by AMS and draw a flowchart to show various decisions that must be made. Can you translate this into a piece of software?
7. What do you see as the future of medical decision making? Will there be more automation or more human centered modes of decision making? Discuss.

References:ii
[1] Makeham M, Dovey S, County M et al (2002) An international taxonomy for errors in general practice: a pilot study. Med Jour Australia 177:68-72
[2] Website for information on cognitive load: http://en.wikipedia.org/wiki/Cognitive_load
[3] Favela, J. Rodriguez, M. Preciado, A. Gonzalez, V.M. (2004) Integrating context-aware public displays into a mobile hospital information system. IEEE Transactions on Information Technology in Biomedicine 8(3):279-286
[4] Skov, M, Hoegh, R (2006) Supporting information access in a hospital ward by a context-aware mobile electronic patient record. Personal and Ubiquitous Computing (Springer-Verlag) 10(4): 205 - 214
[5] Workman, M, Lesser M, Kim, J (2007) An exploratory study of cognitive load in diagnosing patient conditions. International Journal for Quality in Healthcare, 19(3): 127-133, June

Chapter 8: Health Monitoring using Infrastructure-oriented Wireless Networks

Abstract There is considerable interest in using wireless and mobile technologies in health monitoring in diverse environments including homes, assisted living facilities, and nursing homes. In this chapter, we discuss how infrastructure-oriented wireless networks, including commercial cellular/3G and versions of IEEE 802.11 wireless LANs, can be used to support health monitoring in diverse environments. We also present a multi-network architecture to address the reliability requirements of wireless health monitoring.

8.1 Introduction

The comprehensive health monitoring solutions for home healthcare, assisted living care, and nursing home care for stationary and mobile patients can be supported by wireless networks. It can be observed that there has been some progress related to health monitoring using wearable devices and short-range communications. As an increasing number of patients will wear or use communications devices, a comprehensive health monitoring solution can be developed using infrastructure-oriented networks. The use of infrastructure-oriented wireless networks could include cellular type networks (2G, 3G, 4G), wireless LANs, and satellites. The reason these networks are called infrastructure-oriented is that the network components are kept fixed in their locations and the user mobility is supported by handoff or switching to another base station or access point.

Although there are several different types of infrastructure-oriented wireless networks, in this chapter, we focus on cellular/3G and wireless LANs. Cellular/3G networks are commercial and available in most cities in most countries, while wireless LANs are mostly privately owned by individuals and companies. Cellular/3G networks are open to paying subscribers, while wireless LANs are either deployed for employees of a company, individual users at home, or customers at hotels, restaurants and public places. Both cellular/3G and wireless LANs can work outdoors and indoors, although wireless LANs may experience interference from other networks using the same unlicensed ISM bands. Cellular/3G networks use licensed frequency, thus not experiencing interference from other networks which can not use the same frequencies.

The monitoring of patients in homes, assisted living facilities, or nursing homes can be performed by using infrastructure-oriented wireless networks such as wireless LANs [1]. This will allow monitoring for mobile and stationary patients in in-

U. Varshney, *Pervasive Healthcare Computing: EMR/EHR, Wireless and Health Monitoring*, 165
DOI: 10.1007/978-1-4419-0215-3_8,
© Springer Science + Business Media, LLC 2009

door and outdoor environments. Due to its availability, 802.11 WLANs are being used and in some cases, in conjunction with Bluetooth technologies. The cellular/3G networks can also work with Bluetooth integrated in the cell phones. The cellular/3G networks provide dedicated channels and can decline a request for connection if no channels are available. Wireless LANs provide shared access to network bandwidth and the share of bandwidth fluctuates based on the number of active users. This can also add some delays in W-LANs. The bandwidth provided by cellular/3G networks can fluctuate but delays may not be affected so much as the wireless channels are dedicated.

The wireless LANs can be installed quickly by installing access points and connecting them together or to another network. The cost of access points has come down significantly, allowing wireless LANs to be available at lower initial cost. Assuming cellular/3G service can be obtained for the location of monitoring, the initial cost may be low, but certain monthly charges will exist. More work is needed in evaluating the reliability of monitoring using wireless LANs and also by cellular/3G networks.

There has been some work in exploring, designing, testing and implementing infrastructure-oriented wireless networks for health monitoring. A general high-level overview of wireless networks in mobile health can be found in [2]. A survey of wireless networks for health monitoring is presented in [3]. The use of wireless LANs for health monitoring in different scenarios, corresponding requirements and design of network architectures is discussed in [4].

The design and implementation of a prototype for transmitting simplified ECG signals over 802.11 wireless LANs is presented in [5]. A simple algorithm for switching between indoor wireless LAN and outdoor CDMA network for patient monitoring is presented in [6]. The algorithm compares the signal strength between two networks before performing a handoff.

An off-the-shelf implementation of wireless LAN connecting PDAs together in a hospital is described in [7]. The work includes usability, interference testing and security. The authors report that interference with other RF-enabled devices was not found and VPN security was sufficient. The authors also identified that their "killer application" was the need to access blood results [7]. A monitoring of heart rate variability using clothing-embedded transducers transmitting to a PDA and then to a server using wireless LAN is presented in [9]. The PDAs were used as a mobile gateway, which collected information from multiple sensors.

A system that combines Bluetooth and wireless LANs for patient monitoring is described in [11]. The authors propose the use of four different monitoring devices for meeting the diverse requirements of medical staff.

The use of Generalized Packet Radio Service (GPRS) as part of commercial cellular/3G networks for ECG monitoring for arrhythmia is described in [10]. The prototype added GPS location data before transmitting over the network to a remote station for monitoring. The use of wireless application protocol (WAP) over cell phones using GSM data service is shown in [12]. The authorized personnel can view patients' physiological parameters on WAP devices in store-and-forward mode. The use of GSM networks in conjunction with other technologies including GPS and GIS for designing a stray prevention system is shown in [13]. The system is useful for elderly people with dementia and supports four different types of monitoring. Family members or volunteer workers can identify the real-time positions of missing elderly using mobile phone or PDA.

8.2 Networking Requirements of Wireless Health Monitoring

This includes support for a range of monitoring devices, wide coverage, high reliability, low monitoring delays, good scalability and high bit rates, support for confidentiality and privacy, location management, the ability to reach to multiple healthcare professionals, the selection of or adaptation to wireless networks, manageable cognitive load, and use of emerging wireless technologies.

8.2.1 Support for Monitoring Devices

The health monitoring devices are likely to be very diverse in their functionalities and capabilities, such as battery power. This is because wireless health monitoring could involve sensors on-body, implantable devices, wearable devices, portable devices, and/or sensors in the patient environment. These devices must be utilized in terms of power and processing, and must also be matched to the physical conditions of the monitored patients. Therefore, wireless and mobile networks must support a range of monitoring devices. Even a single patient may have more than one type of monitoring device that may require wireless connectivity. In general, certain devices may be more suited to certain networks, such as sensors for Bluetooth networks while hand-held devices for wireless LANs or cellular/3G networks.

8.2.2 Wide Coverage

The coverage requirement for WHM could range from small body area networks to local area networks to wide area networks depending on the distance between monitored patients and the healthcare professionals who need to be notified of the patients' conditions. In general, healthcare professionals are likely to be in the same area or floor for nursing homes, in the same building for assisted living, and in the same city for home-bound and some mobile patients. In some cases of mobile patients, healthcare professionals may be far away and may have to coordinate the necessary help with local medical services and institutions. The coverage should support both fixed and mobile patients. In some cases, the patient mobility could result in uneven distribution of patients, thus making it difficult to perform reliable health monitoring. The monitoring support should also cover patients in both indoor as well as outdoor environment. Some wireless networks, such as satellites, primarily work well in the outdoor environment.

8.2.3 High Reliability

The reliability of wireless networks can be defined as the ability to provide end-to-end wireless health monitoring when needed. Due to the potentially life threatening situations, the reliability of message delivery to healthcare professionals is the most crucial networking requirement of health monitoring. Several factors such as the signal quality variation, failures in the network, and network load may affect such reliability. Although mobile and wireless networks do not inter-operate well due to differences in communications media, protocols, and frequencies, but use of multi-interface devices which can access multiple wireless networks could result in substantial improvement in end-to-end reliability for wireless health monitoring.

For many battery-limited devices, another challenge is to conserve device power while satisfying the reliability requirement of health monitoring. The influencing factors are transmitted power required per message, the number of messages that must be routed, and, routing scheme, which can affect both power requirement and reliability [14].

8.2.4 Low Monitoring Delays

One of the major requirements of WHM is to be able to support message delivery in reasonable time. The network should deliver the messages carrying vital signs within a certain time determined by the level of emergency. The delays could rise substantially under frequent monitoring or for an increased number of monitored patients. One way to support the monitoring delay requirements is to use real-time services provided by some wireless networks such as satellites and cellular networks. Although wireless LANs, such as IEEE 802.11, offer priority for more important packets, these do not support real-time services.

8.2.5 Scalability and High Bit Rates

Scalability is the system's ability to provide performance at a reasonable level with increases in the number of users, distance, applications, bit rate or traffic (Figure 8.1). A single system is unlikely to be scalable with respect to all the parameters. In practice, most systems are not scalable and some are partly scalable with increase in one parameter. For example, some systems may be scalable to number of devices, thus have a place closer to Y axis in Figure 8.1. In practice, the performance of a scalable system may drop, but such degradation is graceful and not extreme.

The design, development and implementation of scalable systems have always been a difficult task and wireless systems are no exceptions. The health monitoring network should scale well in terms of the number of patients. The influencing factors are the bit rate, frequency of monitoring and transmission, and the amount of information per patient. The bit rates should be high enough to support the varying health monitoring traffic. The actual bit rate supported by wireless networks may vary, especially for W-LANs where available bit rate is a function of distance, channel quality and sharing with other users.

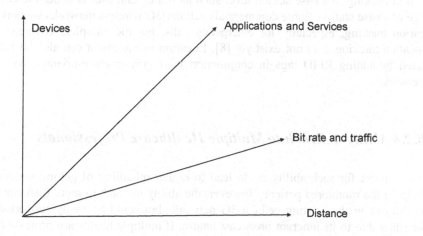

Fig. 8.1 The Dimensions of Scalability

8.2.6 Support for Confidentiality and Privacy

As healthcare information is being transmitted over wireless networks, efforts should be made to keep it confidential and private. This is expected to be the most critical requirements for healthcare administrators and government regulators. Some wireless networks and devices may be more vulnerable to attacks from hackers, who could cause damages ranging from accessing or modifying confidential patient information to attempts for identity theft for potential healthcare benefits. Such challenges should be addressed carefully while selecting a wireless network for health monitoring. Both network layer and application layer security schemes could be deployed to meet the requirements of wireless health monitoring.

8.2.7 Support for Location Management

The location tracking is necessary in WHM to deliver healthcare services, find patients with dementia and other illnesses, and tracking medical supplies. The level of location-awareness varies among wireless networks. W-LANs may support location-tracking at a base station level such as if a certain user is under the coverage of a base station. Some commercials cellular/3G wireless networks support location tracking, especially for emergency calls, but the complete coverage for location tracking does not exist yet [8]. Location management can also be facilitated by adding RFID tags in conjunction with infrastructure-oriented wireless networks.

8.2.8 Ability to Reach to Multiple Healthcare Professionals

The support for such ability could lead to higher reliability of getting necessary help for the monitored patient. However, the ability to reach to more than one HP is difficult in the existing cellular/3G networks but could be easily supported in satellites due to its inherent broadcast nature. If multiple healthcare professionals are in the range, wireless LANs could support this requirement to some extent.

8.2.9 The Selection of or Adaptation to Wireless Networks

The challenge of supporting many requirements of WHM by the existing mobile and wireless networks could become difficult. This can generally be addressed by either the use of existing wireless and mobile networks where selecting the most appropriate ones or adapting to the most easily available ones or creating middleware/application layer protocols to support WHM without requiring a specific wireless and mobile network. Both of these approaches have their advantages and disadvantages. In the first approach, the closest match between requirements and functionalities of available wireless networks may not be satisfactory or may change with time. In the second approach, adding an extra layer of protocols may slow down the monitoring process or add more complexity to monitoring devices.

8.2.10 Manageable Cognitive Load

The health monitoring system should not overwhelm healthcare professionals with a large number of monitoring messages. The computational capabilities of the devices need to be utilized to make intelligent decisions about the patient condition and alerting the healthcare professional only when an anomaly is detected.

8.2.11 Use of Emerging Technologies

This could include the use of emerging and high-potential technologies such as UltraWideBand (UWB) and next generation Bluetooth. For example, UWB uses a wide range of frequency for transmitting low power pulses of signals, while next generation of BT uses higher bit rate with some changes in protocols. As some of these emerging technologies become closer to patients, wireless networks should interwork with these technologies to help extending the range.

8.3. Advantages of Cellular/3G for Health Monitoring

There are several advantages in using cellular/3G networks for wireless health monitoring. To start with, these networks were originally designed for real-time voice communications and wireless data is just one of many services that have been added as the networks have evolved.

8.3.1 Real-time Delivery

Commercial cellular/3G networks, designed for voice communications, provide real-time delivery for carried traffic. So if the wireless health monitoring is done using a voice channel, the monitoring delays would be minimal and thus support-ing the delay requirements of WHM. If the health monitoring is done using non-voice channels or control channels, as also done for SMS, then there may be some delays as the messages are stored-and-forwarded to the destinations. Even in that case, delays would be from few seconds to few minutes. The delay for data ser-vices, such as GPRS, is influenced by the message size, channel rate and the cur-rent network traffic. It may be an interesting study to compare end-to-end moni-toring delay for WHM using voice channels, SMS and GPRS data service.

8.3.2 Wide Coverage

The commercial cellular/3G networks have been able to provide nationwide cov-erage with a few exceptions in some rural or less densely populated areas. Al-though major wireless carriers have coverage in cities and close-by areas, the na-tionwide roaming is achieved by agreements with local and smaller wireless carriers serving smaller areas. Increasingly most countries have commercial cellu-lar/3G networks, although the coverage may be less reliable in some remote areas.

8.3.3 Bandwidth for WHM

As the focus of commercial cellular/3G networks has been individual users, one or more channels are assigned to a user. Such assignment usually results in a band-width ranging from few Kbps to few hundred Kbps per user. In an absolute term, such level may not be great or could even be called broadband, but could support individual monitoring of patients. More work is needed in measuring blocking of health monitoring traffic due to temporary lack of channels in some locations.

8.3.4 Ability to Work with other Wireless Technologies

Although commercial cellular/3G networks are known to have several different and incompatible standards, cellular/3G phones could work with other wireless technologies such as Bluetooth or sensor networks (Figure 8.2). This becomes possible as the phones are being added with additional adapters. This will allow cellular/3G networks to act as a backbone technology for many wireless health monitoring scenarios where a personal area network or a short-range wireless technology is employed for direct monitoring.

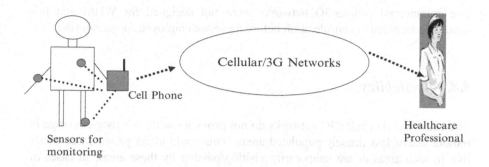

Fig. 8.2 Cellular/3G Networks Working with Sensor Networks

8.3.5 Widely Used Technology

People, especially many patients and healthcare professionals, have been using cellular/3G technologies for some time and there appears to be a considerable degree of comfort in using these technologies. This could be an important factor in selection and adoption of cellular/3G networks for wireless health monitoring.

8.3.6 Secure

The commercial cellular/3G networks use strong encryption and generally known to have a very high-level of secure communications over wireless links. Although not all, but some of cellular/3G networks, such as GSM, also authenticate their users before any communications could start. This could provide a high level of security for wireless health monitoring.

8.3.7 Support for Location Management

The commercial cellular/3G networks support location management. This is an important feature for health monitoring as knowing the patient's location will allow the delivery of needed help. This will also be helpful for cases when a patient is lost due to dementia or other cognitive problems.

8.4 Limitations of Cellular/3G for WHM

The commercial cellular/3G networks were not designed for WHM and this should be included in consideration before these are employed for monitoring.

8.4.1 Availability

The commercial cellular/3G networks do not provide usable or strong coverage in remote and/or less densely populated areas. This could affect patients that either live in such areas or are temporarily visiting/passing by these areas. In cases of emergency, this could become a major problem.

8.4.2 Presence of Dead-spots

It is known that due to various radio related problems, cellular/3G networks exhibit the presence of dead-spots (or cold-spots) where coverage is poor or unusable (Figure 8.3) Although, many enhancements have been added to commercial cellular/3G networks over the years, the time and location-dependent presence of such spots still exists.

8.4.3 Reliability Challenges

The reliability of commercial cellular/3G networks is not widely known. When failures occur, many times people misinterpret the lack of access due to network overload and not due to failure of a base station or some other network component. In practice, a range of network components could fail affecting coverage and the reliability of wireless health monitoring. In addition, the network performance will also affect the reliability of patient monitoring. More specifically, error rates and handoff failures by the network in the middle of monitoring could negatively affect the reliability of health monitoring. It is known that cellular/3G networks may also experience call dropping of several percent, thus bringing down the reliability level not acceptable for emergency messages. Certainly, more work is needed in evaluating the reliability in a range of monitoring scenarios involving cellular/3G networks.

8.4.4 Lack of Broadcast/Multicast

Having the ability to multicast or broadcast is useful for reliable WHM as it allows the health monitoring information to reach to multiple healthcare professionals. However, as commercial cellular/3G networks are designed for one-to-one communications, such ability is difficult, not impossible though, to implement at the network level. In cases, where such ability is crucial, application-layer multicast, with additional protocols, will have to be designed and utilized.

8.4.5 Pricing

The commercial cellular/3G networks offer two types of pricing: the per-minute charges and the charges by data volume with an additional minimum charge. Although there are carriers who offer unlimited minutes in some locations to some users, in general minutes-based pricing will make continuous monitoring difficult to support. The second type of pricing may be more suitable for wireless health monitoring. However, the recurring monthly charges for cellular/3G could be an obstacle in wider deployment and adoption of wireless health monitoring.

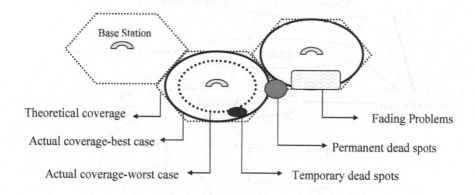

Fig. 8.3 Coverage Problems in Cellular Networks

8.4.6 The Impact of Commercial Traffic

Currently there is a lack of priority for different traffic, except for national emergency cases, and thus a first come first served allocation will allow a voice call to continue while WHM traffic may have to wait and keep retrying. The impact of other commercial traffic could be very negative for WHM traffic. Work is needed in creating high priority (or guaranteed) bandwidth allocation for WHM traffic.

8.5 Advantages of W-LANs in Health Monitoring

Many healthcare applications require reliable monitoring of patients such as those in a hospital or nursing home. Currently in a typical nursing home in the US, a patient is observed by a nurse or staff one to few times an hour, however if a patient is experiencing chest pain or heart attack while in the bathroom alone, the required help may not come in time. To improve this situation, health monitoring can be done using infrastructure-oriented wireless networks such as most of the existing and emerging wireless LANs [1]. This will allow monitoring for mobile and stationary patients in indoor and outdoor environments (Figure 8.4).

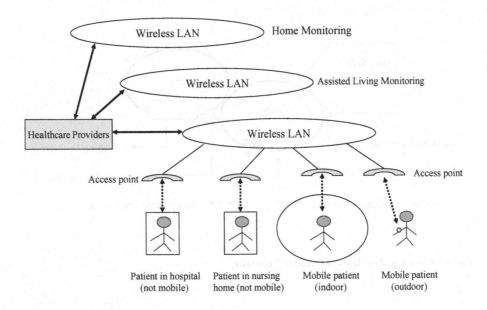

Fig. 8.4 Health Monitoring using Wireless LANs

There are many major issues related to health monitoring using infrastructure-oriented wireless LANs. These include the service area and signal reception, throughput and bit rates, number of patients that can be supported, co-located operation and interference issues, signal transmission from patients to access points, monitoring delays, location accuracy, protocol, and reliability of health monitoring using wireless LANs. In the next few paragraphs, we discuss these issues one by one.

8.5.1 Bit Rates for WHM

The throughput, or actual number of bits that can be transmitted after subtracting overhead and retransmission, decreases with an increasing distance between patients and access points, so either a higher number of access points per wireless LAN or a higher bit rate wireless LAN should be employed. The different versions of WLANs will offer different throughput, which is about 30-40% lower than the maximum possible bit rate. The number of patients that can be supported by an access point will depend on the bit rate, frequency of monitoring, and the amount of information per patient that needs to be sent every time.

8.5.2 Transmission from Patients to AP

Another major issue is how signals would be transmitted from patients to wireless access points. This will depend on if patients can wear or carry devices with WLAN adapter cards that transmit signals to a base station. If not, then for every few patients, one device with an adapter card can proxy and transmit signals to one or more access points. This will be useful if patients wear devices with short-range of signal transmission. The device usability and accessibility issues must be addressed along with size and portability of devices that must be carried.

8.5.3 Support for Mobile Patients

The health monitoring system will support both fixed and mobile patients (and also patients that are fixed sometime and mobile sometime). The mobility of patients will create uneven number of users under different access points. This will affect both throughput and delays for health monitoring. For such cases, prioritized transmission could be employed for patient with emergency signal. To support mobility, most wireless LANs use synchronization for finding and staying with a WLAN, power management for periodic sleep and letting a device sleep without missing any message, and association and re-association for joining a network and moving from one access point to another. A device scans all the possible frequency channels and looks for a beacon signal for the network it wants to join.

8.5.4 Location Management

Health monitoring does require location management of patient in addition to the transmission of their vital signs over infrastructure-oriented wireless LANs. To support this, individual access points can maintain a list of currently supported patients. This would support location management with an accuracy equal to the size of its coverage. This may be enough for some applications, however, access points can combine other location management technologies such as RFID (radio frequency identification) for better tracking of patients.

8.5.5 Access Protocols

For medium access control (MAC), most wireless LANs use Collision Sense Multiple Access with Collision Avoidance (CSMA/CA) as opposed to CSMA/CD where collision detection is required. The medium access control (MAC) frame contains destination MAC address, source MAC address, data, and cyclical redundancy control (CRC) for frame checking. In wireless LANs, once the channel is free from the previous transmissions, devices can attempt to access it for their transmissions. As part of the MAC protocols, different devices are required to wait different amount of time after the channel is free before transmitting (so if you have to wait less, you in effect have a higher priority). The waiting time (or inter frame space) is dependent on what you have to transmit (such as acknowledgement, Clear-To-Send, poll response will be transmitted with higher priority or lower waiting time-called short inter frame space). This kind of reduced waiting, or effectively a higher priority, can also be used to support transmission of abnormal or emergency signals. This could reduce the total end-to-end delays for health monitoring.

8.6 Limitations of W-LANs for WHM

Wireless LANs were not originally designed for health monitoring applications, but the wider deployment and lower cost have made them an attractive choice.

However, there are challenges of limited coverage, varying levels of security, variable delays, interference from other networks, lack of reliability and multicast.

8.6.1 Limited Coverage

The service area of most access points in wireless LANs is limited to about 100 meters, but is affected by mobility, obstacles, and many problems. The range (or service area) is also affected by the frequency used in WLANs. The signal strength can be weakened by 30-90% as it passes through doors, walls, and windows depending on the material and construction employed. Thus these problems will reduce the coverage area of WLANs indoor. And, the outdoor coverage may be impacted by moving vehicles, other WLANs and trees. To increase the coverage of a wireless LAN, the number of access points can be increased, resulting in higher initial cost. Another issue is the availability of wireless links between patients and access points. The link quality varies over space and time due to attenuation (power loss) caused to a signal as it passes through walls, doors, windows, and humans. The power loss and/or interference can cause links to fail momentarily or completely. So the full connectivity or 100% availability cannot be assumed even if everything else is fine. It is very difficult to measure the pattern of link availability as the movement of objects changes the interference type and level. Even when coverage exists, the links may be unusable due to one or more fading problems as links alternate between usable and unusable states.

8.6.2 Security

W-LANs are more vulnerable due to the use of unlicensed spectrum and the use of weaker encryption makes it even worse. In many ways, the wireless LANs are not suited to the high security and confidentiality requirements of wireless health monitoring unless a stronger encryption can be deployed along with authentication of patients to be monitored.

8.6.3 Monitoring Delays

Another issue related to health monitoring using wireless LANs is the monitoring delays that may be created by access points and WLAN protocols. It should be noted that almost all WLANs were designed for data-type traffic where delays were not critical. The delays occur as patients will have to wait for transmission and can be reduced selectively using prioritized transmission. However, such problems will affect the quality of health monitoring. The delays could rise substantially, if many more patients happen to be under the coverage of the same access point due to locational restrictions or due to mobility.

8.6.4 Co-located Networks

One major issue in infrastructure-oriented WLANs is the need to allow co-located network operation where multiple WLANs may exist in the same or nearby location. The multiple WLANs will create additional interference for one another due to the use of same ISM band. This may also reduce the amount of bandwidth usable for WHM. Although co-located operation affects different wireless LANs differently based on the physical layer transmission and the choice of ISM band used, in general the throughput is reduced due to an increased ISM interference. No coordinating body exists yet to register all WLANs in all locations. Also, due to reflection of a signal from other objects, the receiver gets multiple copies of a signal. These copies are slightly shifted in phase (time), so overlapping may occur, which makes it hard to decode a signal. The multi-path interference is the biggest challenge to high-speed data communications as bits become smaller and even a slight shift of phase can cause significant interference. This is a problem for higher bit rate WLANs. Also, as ISM band is used in wireless LANs, interference from unlicensed spectrum radio, microwave ovens, or radar transmitters may also exist affecting the usability and coverage of infrastructure-oriented wireless LANs for health monitoring.

8.6.5 Reliability

The major issue is the reliability of health monitoring using WLANs. The reliability here is affected by several factors: coverage and signal strength, available bit rate and prioritized transmission, delay performance, and failure of access points and interconnection architecture. The first three factors have been addressed in the preceding paragraphs, we now address failure of access points and interconnection architecture. To reduce the impact of access point failures, we propose that both overlapping and back-up access points be deployed. This will improve coverage in normal cases and continued coverage even when one or more failures occur. The access points can be interconnected in a grid of wireless LANs using mesh-based interconnection. The mesh, due to its rich interconnection pattern or high redundancy of links, is highly reliable interconnection architecture.

The protocol for health monitoring using WLANs should involve the following steps:

1. Patient's devices to locate and join an access point
2. Patient's device to measure vital signs (if above or below normal, transmit a signal to access point using higher priority. If matches a pattern or highly above or below normal, transmit an "emergency" signal to the access point using highest priority)
3. Access point to route the message to one or more healthcare providers along with past vital signs (from a database) and the current location of the patient.

Also, the number of patients that can be monitored under every access point can be limited to provide both improved and reliable health monitoring services. These limits can be derived, differently for multiple versions of 802.11 WLANs, based on the traffic generated (frequency of monitoring and packets per monitoring event) and the delay requirements.

8.6.6 Multicast Support

Health monitoring would need group communication among users. The most efficient way to support this requirement is wireless multicast, where the information exchange among users is performed and membership of a group is maintained. As mobile users move to different locations or leave the group or new users join the group, the membership information is updated for network traffic routing. To support multicast-based health monitoring in wireless LANs, the followings are necessary: (a) identifying the multicast requirements of health monitoring, and (b) modeling and evaluating the overhead caused due to protocol modifications. Based on the current locations of healthcare professionals, some of the access points could become part of the multicast tree in transmitting healthcare information to multiple destinations or healthcare professionals.

8.7 Comparison of Cellular/3G and Wireless LANs

Based on the advantages and disadvantages presented in the last few sections, a comparison between cellular/3G and wireless LANs is shown in Table 8.1. This will help in selecting the best choice to meet the requirements of specific wireless health monitoring environment.

Table 8.1 Qualitative Comparison of Cellular/3G and Wireless LANs

Attribute	Cellular/3G	WLANs
Support for a range of monitoring devices	Yes	Yes
Wide coverage	Yes, but some dead spots and unreliable coverage areas	No, additional infrastructure needed
High reliability	No, more work is needed	No, many challenges must be addressed
Low monitoring delays	Yes, with real-time delivery	No, variable and high delays (but priority could be used)
Scalability and high bit rates	Sufficient for WHM	Sufficient for WHM
Confidentiality and privacy	Yes, using strong encryption	No, needs work to meet WHM requirements
Location Management	Yes	Yes, base station level
	Could also work with other locational technologies	Could also work with other locational technologies
Ability to reach to multiple HPs	No, lack of multicast	Yes, with support for multicast
Cost	Low initial cost but recurring monthly charges (so high overall cost)	Some initial cost but little to no monthly charges (so low overall cost)
Use of emerging technologies	Yes	Yes
	Could also provide backbone to other wireless networks including W-LANs	

8.8 Reliability for Wireless Health Monitoring

The reliability could broadly include the reliability of wireless infrastructure, reliability of monitoring devices and sensors, reliability of information collection, reliability of information transmission, and reliability of healthcare professionals' devices. Here the focus is on the reliability of wireless networks and infrastructure.

Wireless health monitoring requires a highly reliable network access anywhere anytime. One way to create reliable access is to utilize multiple wireless networks that may be available at a given location. The vital signs and environmental variables can be divided in several packets, transmitted over wireless networks, and aggregated before being delivered to one or more healthcare professionals, who could also access/receive stored information on the patient. In addition to vital signs, environmental variables such as room temperature, humidity, and patient's activity-exercise, food, discussion, resting, walking can also be transmitted over multiple networks and combined on the other side by a health monitoring environment. This reliable wireless network architecture will allow health monitoring to work even under:

- Failure in networks: when base stations, mobile devices, or databases experience failure
- Coverage limitations: when cellular wireless networks experience coverage problems
- Intermittent access: when a device is unable to access a network continuously

The reliable wireless network architecture will allow users to overcome time and/or location-sensitive dis-connectivity or intermittent connectivity problems and failures in one network by switching to another wireless network. To further increase the level of reliability, fault-tolerance can be introduced at network, device, data (replication) and applications level. The reliability enhancements may also include design and deployment of a grid of wireless LANs, and combining WLANs and commercial cellular networks. A possible architecture is shown in Figure 8.5, where health monitoring devices can access and switch among cellular/3rd Generation, wireless LANs, ad-hoc wireless networks, and sensors-based networks. We assume (a) devices have the intelligence to sense presence of multiple wireless networks, (b) local characteristics of individual wireless networks are available and can be used in deciding which network to switch to, and, (c) devices have the hardware to switch among multiple networks.

Each of the networks may have its own complexity in terms of total bandwidth, usable bandwidth, coverage and reliability, required power level for transmission, priorities for access and transmission, and, any protocol specific requirements. For example, satellites may have wider outdoor coverage; however the indoor coverage is not reliable. Wireless LANs can offer inexpensive network access in Industrial, Medical and Scientific (ISM) band, which is also unlicensed for lots of other use. Cellular/3G networks offer high quality access, but the cost for access may be too high for continuous health monitoring. Also, the location and time-dependent dead spots may affect the quality of comprehensive health monitoring. Sensors and RFID are very short range and will be needed in large numbers to provide any reasonable coverage. Although individually a single wireless network may not be able to provide reliability, coverage, and networking resource necessary to allow highly reliable health monitoring, but the ability to access and switch among multiple networks may create a fault-tolerant architecture with richer set of resources, capable of overcoming multiple problems.

In the next few years, Fourth Generation (4G) wireless networks could emerge allowing users to access multiple wireless networks without manually switching from network to network. Additional research is needed in estimating the overhead of multi-network access including handoffs among networks, processing overhead of dividing and aggregating vital signs and related information, and the level of end-to-end reliability achieved in several different variations of the architecture.

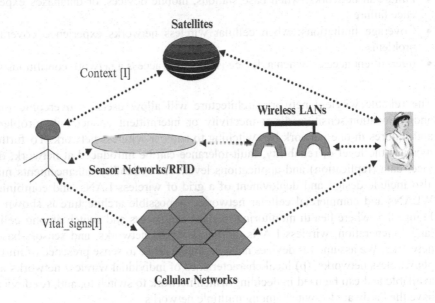

Fig. 8.5 Improving Infrastructure Reliability by Using Multiple Networks

8.9 Other Networking Considerations

In addition to network reliability, more work is also needed in managing network traffic and supporting performance considerations [15].

8.9.1 Managing Network Traffic

In practice, wireless health monitoring could generate considerable traffic, especially if a large number of patients are sharing a wireless network, such as a wireless LAN in a nursing home. To address this, the health monitoring traffic can be managed at multiple places.

1. Source device: This includes managing the frequency of monitoring, the number and frequency of vital signs, the information per packet, the number of gen-

erated packets, and compression to reduce the traffic offered to a wireless network.

2. Wireless network: This includes use of priority, use of both live and stored information, admission control, use of incentives for co-operation, and use of routing scheme to support reliability of message delivery.

3. Health professional's device: This includes filtering of duplicated information, use of live vs stored information, and use of context-awareness.

8.9.2 Performance Considerations

As stated before, not all wireless networks have characteristics that would meet all the requirements of wireless health monitoring. To show the suitability and effectiveness of individual or multiple wireless networks working together, work is needed in performance evaluation. The following metrics can be used in the modeling and measuring the effectiveness of network infrastructure for health monitoring:

1. The reduction in monitoring delays and network traffic by using stored and live information

2. The accessibility of health monitoring system (fraction of time) to measure reliability

3. The number of incorrect decisions (incorrect context, cognitive load of providers)

Some research challenges in wireless networks for health monitoring are:

1. Deriving protocols to decide when and how to transmit differential changes in vital signs by wireless networks and nominal values by accessing stored knowledge, and when to switch from one mode (pure wireless network transmission) to mixed mode (use of stored information combined with differential traffic over wireless networks)

2. Measuring the amount of overhead in traffic management strategies

3. Evaluating the impact of traffic management, such as information integration on the scalability of wireless health monitoring system.

8.10 Future

In the future, infrastructure-oriented wireless networks including both commercial cellular/3G as well as wireless LANs will play a major role in wireless health monitoring. Several things that will help in this dominant role are higher bit rates and changes in the protocols, improved reliability of monitoring, and reduced cost of monitoring.

One is the bit rate per user that would need to be increased to support higher-end applications. To address the demands of future wireless LANs, IEEE High Throughput Task Force (802.11n) is considering ways to increase bit rates to several hundred Mbps. Even if this is shared among multiple patients, bit rate per user would still be sufficient to support wireless health monitoring. Also, the number of patients that can be monitored under every access point/base station can be limited to provide both improved and reliable health monitoring services. These limits can be derived for multiple versions of 802.11 WLANs, based on the traffic generated (frequency of monitoring and packets per monitoring event) and the delay requirements. More work can also be done in modifying WLAN protocols to suit healthcare applications. This could include support for higher priority for healthcare data, improved security and privacy, higher bit rates, and, support for both continuous and in-frequent (as needed) monitoring. Additionally, the support for allocating lower frequency spectrum for health monitoring will be very helpful as low power monitoring devices would be able to transmit.

The cost of health monitoring could reduce for infrastructure-oriented networks with continued reduction in the initial cost of installing wireless LANs and by better traffic-based pricing from cellular/3G networks. To support widespread use of WHM, the government can provide subsidies or financial support to allow continuous monitoring over cellular/3G networks, which may not be otherwise affordable for monitoring for people with limited income, including retirees and older patients. Wireless carriers and manufactures may also offer programs to support certain demographics or type of patients in their financial needs for health monitoring.

The future research should address how to improve the reliability of health monitoring under varying coverage of wireless LANs, wireless link variations, and access point failures. The reliability of wireless LANs based monitoring can be improved by using multiple access points that could provide overlapping/back-up coverage in cases of access point failure. The work should also address commercial cellular/3G networks. The development of hardware which can support multi-network access will also be very helpful in enhancing the achievable reliability of health monitoring.

Questions
1.   Suggest and discuss several ways to improve reliability of infrastructure-oriented wireless networks.
2.   Discuss how the cost of monitoring can be estimated for cellular/3G and wireless LANs and discuss how it will affect the adoption of wireless health monitoring.

3. Why the ability to reach to more than one healthcare professional is necessary in wireless health monitoring? How can we add multicast support in infrastructure-oriented wireless networks?
4. How to manage lower delays in wireless health monitoring?
5. What level of location accuracy can be obtained in infrastructure-oriented wireless networks? What improvements are possible by adding RFID to these networks?
6. Show an example where infrastructure-oriented wireless networks could work with other wireless technologies.
7. Can infrastructure-oriented wireless networks act as a backbone network for other networks including other infrastructure-oriented wireless networks?
8. Discuss two factors that will seriously impact your decision to select an infrastructure-oriented wireless network for wireless health monitoring.

REFERENCES
[1] Varshney U (2003) The status and future of 802.11-based WLANs. IEEE Computer, 36(6):102-105, June
[2] Guest Editorial (2004) M-health: beyond seamless mobility and global wireless healthcare connectivity. IEEE Transactions on IT in Biomedicine, 8(4):405-414, December
[3] Varshney U (2007) Pervasive healthcare and wireless patient monitoring. ACM/Springer Journal on Mobile Networks and Applications (MONET), 12(2-3):113-127, March
[4] Varshney U (2006) Patient monitoring using infrastructure-oriented wireless LANs. Int. J. on Electronic Healthcare, 2(2):149-163
[5] Tejero-Calado et.al (2005) IEEE 802.11 ECG monitoring system. Proc. 27th Annu. Int. Conf. IEEE Eng. Med. Biol. Soc., 7139-7142
[6] Ko W, Jeong E, Kim S, Cho H, Kim W (2003) Implementation of a handover between wireless LANs and public cellular CDMA network for a portable patient monitoring system. In Proc. EMBS Asia-Pacific Conference on Biomedical Engineering, 98-99
[7] Turner P, Milne G, Kubitscheck M, Penman I, Turner S (2005) Implementing a wireless network of PDAs in a hospital setting. Pervasive and Ubiquitous Computing, 9:209-217
[8] FCC Enhanced 911(www.fcc.gov/e911)
[9] Jovanov E, O'Donnel A, Morgan A, Priddy B, Hormigo R (2002) Prolonged telemetric monitoring of heart rate variability using wireless intelligent sensors and a mobile gateway. In Proc. Second Joint IEEE EMBS/BMES Conference, 1875-1876
[10] Liszka K, Mackin M, Lichter M, York D, Pillai D, Rosenbaum D (2004) Keeping a beat on the heart. IEEE Pervasive Computing Magazine, 42-49, Oct-Dec
[11] Yu S, Cheng J (2005) A wireless physiological signal monitoring system with integrated bluetooth and WiFi technologies. Proc. 27th Annu. Int. Conf. IEEE Eng. Med. Biol. Soc. 2203-2206
[12] Hung K, Zhang Y-T (2003) Implementation of a WAP-based telemedicine system for patient monitoring. IEEE Trans. Inf. Technol. Biomed, 7(2):101-107, June
[13] Lin C, Chiu M, Hsiao C, Lee R, Tsai Y (2006) Wireless health care service system for elderly with dementia. IEEE Trans. Inf. Technol. Biomed, 10(2): 696-704,October
[14] Varshney U, Sneha S (2006) Patient monitoring using ad hoc wireless networks: reliability and power management. IEEE Communications Magazine, 44(4): 49-55, April
[15] Varshney U (2006) Managing wireless health monitoring for patients with disabilities. IEEE IT Professional, 8(6):12-16, Nov.-Dec.

Chapter 9: Ad Hoc Networks for Health Monitoring

Abstract In cases where the coverage of infrastructure-oriented wireless networks such as cellular/3G or wireless LANs is not available or reliable, ad hoc networks can be used to support wireless health monitoring. This chapter focuses on ad hoc networks in wireless health monitoring. However, the use of ad hoc networks does introduce several interesting challenges including reliability, power management and routing. These challenges are discussed and several solutions are proposed.

9.1 Introduction

In most cases, health monitoring will be done by infrastructure-oriented wireless networks such as commercial cellular/3G networks or wireless LANs. But in some cases, either the coverage of wireless network is not available, or the coverage is available but the network can not be accessed due to a lack of available bandwidth. Even with attempts to improve the coverage by several technical enhancements including overlapping base stations, however, some parts of buildings, especially the isolated and corner areas, may have spotty coverage. Also, in some cases, the coverage of the infrastructure-oriented networks fluctuates with time or location. Finally, there may be one or more failures in infrastructure-oriented networks, resulting in access problems. Here are several more problems in supporting health monitoring using infrastructure-oriented wireless networks: (a) short range and limited power capabilities of most patient devices, (b) lack of interoperability among multiple wireless LANs, (c) considerable interference in ISM bands from multiple sources, (d) varying capacity of infrastructure-oriented wireless networks, and, (e) lack of application-specific priority for transmission of emergency signals. These problems and restrictions could result in many cases and scenarios where continuous health monitoring is not possible and/or emergency signals may not be transmitted from a patient to healthcare providers. For these situations, health monitoring can be achieved by using ad hoc wireless networks, formed among patients' devices that can transmit vital signs over a short-range [1, 2].

In practice, three configurations of wireless networks are possible for health monitoring: (a) the end-to-end configuration involving only infrastructure networks, (b) the end-to-end configuration involving only ad hoc networks, and (c) the end-to-end configuration involving a combination of infrastructure networks and ad hoc networks. We refer to these networks as pure infrastructure, pure ad hoc and hy-

U. Varshney, *Pervasive Healthcare Computing: EMR/EHR, Wireless and Health Monitoring*, 189
DOI: 10.1007/978-1-4419-0215-3_9,
© Springer Science + Business Media, LLC 2009

brid configurations. We envision that ad hoc networks would supplement or extend the range of other wireless networks. In practice, it is unlikely that the end-to-end network for health monitoring would be pure ad hoc. Therefore, the wireless monitoring network configuration is likely to be hybrid, including a combination of infrastructure and ad hoc wireless networks.

9.1.1 Ad Hoc Networks for Health Monitoring

Unlike infrastructure-oriented wireless networks, where network components are kept fixed and user mobility is supported by handoff or switching to another access point/base station, ad hoc networks rely on mobile devices acting as routers. Thus communications to a destination is possible by finding a path from the source consisting of one or more devices acting as routers (hops). Due to limited power, efficiency or power conservation is an important challenge. For a given distance, multi-hop ad hoc networks are more power efficient than large single hop ad hoc network due to square relationship between power and distance. For example, to cover 4 unit of distance, a 4-hop network will involve 4 units of power, while single hop network for the same distance will require 16 units of power.

The information on vital signs of a patient can be transmitted to another nearby patient and so on, thus increasing the chance that vital signs are picked up by a healthcare professional on his/her device. A possible scenario is shown in Figure 9.1. Here the ranges of patient devices are shown in dotted circles, while ranges of other routing devices in solid lines. For a device to route your packet, that device has to be in your range to receive the packet in the first place.

This creation of ad hoc wireless networks among patients and devices to allow for movement of sensor information would require wireless routing to allow for information to reach to a healthcare provider. More specifically, as shown in Figure 9.1, the information from device D_2 is routed to D_1, which then routes it to R_i and then R_i sends it to HP_1. The information also travels from D_2 is routed to D_3, which then routes it to R_k and then to R_j which then sends it to HP_1 and HP_2. This example shows how reliable transmission of health information can be achieved using ad hoc networks.

With mobility of patient and devices, the topology of ad hoc networks may change with time. Thus the future transmission of health information may follow a different path to healthcare professionals based on available connectivity, which may be heavily influenced by the coverage and current location of devices.

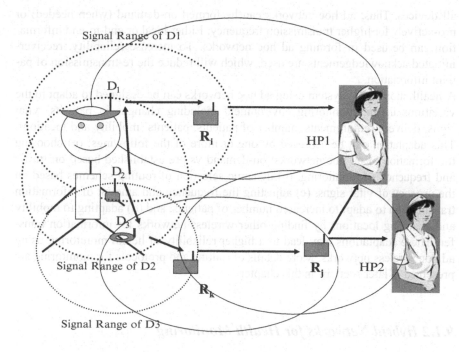

D1, 2, 3: Health monitoring devices

    Ri, j, k: Routing devices

    HP: Healthcare professional

Fig. 9.1 Using Ad Hoc Networks for Health Monitoring

Unlike general-purpose wireless networks, the efficiency of networking operation
is not the major criterion, but the reliability, speed, and error free transmission of
critical information must be supported. The ad hoc networks can be formed on-
demand as needed among health monitoring devices or can be formed in advance
for faster transmission of patient information. Also, the duration of ad hoc networks can be short-lived to support any infrequent transmissions or long-lived if
continuous monitoring is needed. This must be subject to the power levels of
monitoring devices. Multi-hop wireless ad hoc networks are formed between patient and healthcare professionals using the co-operation of other devices acting as
routers. If no nearby device is found, stronger signal must be transmitted from a
patient's device to increase the chances of reception by a far-away device. Multiple way to form and maintain ad hoc networks include keeping track of devices
that are in range using a periodic beacon signal, last received message in a certain
time, or periodic refreshing (updating) of current neighbors in a routing table for

all devices. Thus, ad hoc networks can be formed on-demand (when needed) or pro-actively for higher transmission frequency. Either local or end-to-end information can be used in forming ad hoc networks. To increase reliability, receiver-initiated acknowledgements are used, which will reduce the re-transmission of patient information.

A health monitoring system using ad hoc networks can be designed to adapt to the variations in the monitoring environment including changes in patients' vital signs, delivery requirements, number of patients, patients' mobility and locations. This adaptation can be achieved by one or more of the followings: (a) choosing the formation of ad hoc networks: on-demand vs pre-established based on traffic and frequency of monitoring, (b) dynamic selection of routing schemes based on the urgency of vital signs, (c) adjusting the frequency and amount of information transmission to adapt to increased number of patients, and (d) adapting to mobility and changing locations by finding other wireless networks for information transfer. These adaptations may lead to a higher reliability of health monitoring using ad hoc wireless networks. More details of routing and protocols for monitoring are presented in later sections in this chapter.

9.1.2 Hybrid Networks for Health Monitoring

Several recent studies have proposed, utilized, and showed the usefulness of infrastructure and ad hoc wireless networks in health monitoring [4-8]. This includes CodeBlue, which uses sensor networks and wireless devices in ad hoc networks to create several services, including emergency services, for healthcare environment [4]. This study shows the effectiveness of ad hoc wireless networks with wireless vital sign monitors and a triage application [4]. Also, a prototype for trauma patients is based on measuring vital signs using sensor nodes in an ad hoc network [5]. Ad hoc wireless networks have also been utilized in weight monitoring and wellness management [8]. Certainly more work is needed to support networks of medical sensors. There are several special characteristics, such as low power requirements and asymmetric traffic from medical sensors, which should be included in the design for such networks. A new medium access control protocol for medical sensors in a personal area networking environment can be found in [9].

The network configuration which can provide wireless monitoring support using a combination of wireless networks is shown in Figure 9.2. The configuration includes infrastructure-oriented wireless LANs that support transmission to healthcare professionals using access points. When there is a connectivity problem, the vital signs may be transmitted using ad hoc networks in one or more hops. The two different types of body area networks (BANs), formed by health monitoring sensors and devices that range from a group of sensors, wearable and portable monitors, include intra-BAN and inter-BAN. The intra-BANs are formed among devices on the same patient, while inter-BAN(s) involve communications among devices on different patients and healthcare professionals. We envision that some of the inter-BANs and intra-BANs are ad hoc wireless networks formed among sensors and monitoring devices [4]. It should be noted that the topology of this network is also subject to change with patient and device mobility. Although devices in intra-BAN may not be very mobile, the patient mobility will affect the distance and inter-BAN links. So similar to pure ad hoc networks, hybrid networks are also subject to some complexity in maintaining network connectivity with time.

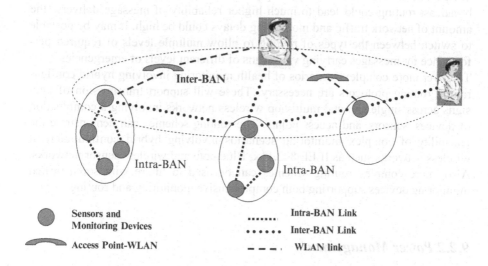

BAN: Body Area Network

Fig. 9.2 Use of Ad Hoc Networks to Support Intra-BAN and Inter-BAN

9.2 Challenges for Wireless Health Monitoring

There are many challenges in ad hoc wireless networks for health monitoring, including routing of monitoring messages with changes in network connectivity and user locations, power management, and reliability of monitoring. These are not necessarily independent challenges as routing will be affected by power management, while reliability will be poor if the chosen routing scheme does not deliver health monitoring messages due to network connectivity and/or power restrictions.

9.2.1 Routing

Several routing schemes, which differ in how messages are routed to a destination, can be considered. Each of these schemes brings its own complexity, overhead and performance in terms of reliability of message delivery and end-to-end delays. The impact of patient mobility, limited device range and failures of routing devices is also likely to be very different on the reliability of these routing schemes. For example, unicast routing will have the worst performance if an intermediate device has failed, moved or is simply not co-operative. While multicast and broadcast routing could lead to much higher reliability of message delivery, the amount of network traffic and monitoring delays could be high. It may be possible to switch between the types of routing to allow multiple levels of required performance for messages carrying vital-signs of different levels of emergencies.

To cover more complex scenarios of health monitoring involving hybrid configuration, routing protocols are necessary. These will support transmission of vital signs across single hop and multi-hop wireless networks involving a combination of devices, sensors, and access points. The routing schemes can demonstrate the feasibility of complex monitoring scenarios involving hybrid configuration of wireless networks such as IEEE 802.11x, Bluetooth and wireless sensor networks. Also, more complex routing schemes can be used in future with sophisticated monitoring devices supporting both comprehensive monitoring and routing.

9.2.2 Power Management

There are additional challenges that must be addressed in transmission over ad hoc wireless networks. These challenges include power management and reliable transmission. Power management has been an important issue in ad hoc networks, however, in health monitoring, it becomes even more important as the transmitted power can influence both the ability of a patient device to transmit monitoring signals as well as the end-to-end routing of these signals [3]. Also, if a patient's device has been involved in the routing of many prior messages from other patients, it may not have sufficient power left when it needs to transmit its own signals. Therefore, power conservation is necessary for such devices, and can be realized by minimizing the frequency and the number of vital signs. Also, the vital signs can be coded differentially to reduce the number of bits that are generated and transmitted in a message.

9.2.3 Reliability

Possible enhancements for improving the reliability of monitoring messages include (i) increased power transmission for improving the chances of finding co-operating devices or a healthcare professional, (ii) multiple retransmissions and hop-by-hop acknowledgements, (iii) increasing the number of co-operating devices (including fixed devices) and healthcare professionals, (iv) transmission of differential value of vital signs, and, (v) use of multiple ad hoc networks [1]. The co-operation of other devices for helping in the routing of monitoring messages in one or more ad hoc networks can be achieved by offering incentives for routing. These could include certain credits for routing which can be used for reducing nursing home expenses, for membership in ad hoc networks when needed, and for prioritized routing of their messages. In some cases, the co-operation of other devices can be made as a requirement for a patient to be in a nursing home or hospital.

9.3 Existing Ad Hoc Networks

There are several possible wireless networks, including both personal area networks, such as Bluetooth and wireless LANs such as 802.11, which can also run in ad hoc mode. Even as an example of simple implementation without priority, there are some problems that must be addressed including the range of ad hoc networks and bit rates of ad hoc networks. The range of existing wireless ad hoc networks, such as Bluetooth is 1-100 meters, based on the type of device and transmitted power. The bit rates offered are likely to be in few hundred Kbps to tens of Mbps. Both range and bit rates could be adequate for health monitoring applications, if frequency of health monitoring is kept low with limited number of monitored patients.

For use of Bluetooth as an ad hoc network for health monitoring, there are other limitations as the number of active users (patients) per piconet is limited to 8, one of which must be master device managing communications within and in some cases to other piconet where it is a member in non-master role. This limit of active devices will affect the total number of patients that can be monitored if Bluetooth is used. The use of multiple piconets for health monitoring is shown in Figure 9.3, where a device acts as a master device in one piconet to forward information from other piconets, where it is serving as a non-master device. This allows the information to travel from a patient to healthcare professional across multiple piconets until another network such as wireless LAN or HP device can be found. Each piconet uses its own sequence of frequency hopping, thus avoiding interference to some extent. However, if several piconets exist in an area, then interference in ISM band could limit the number of types of vital signs that can be transmitted for monitored patients. Also, Bluetooth enforces power control by dividing users among three types, which could affect the range of health monitoring. In theory, these power limits could be matched to the role of patient monitoring devices, routing devices and healthcare professional devices.

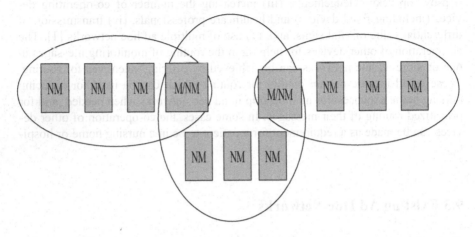

M: Master, NM: Non-master

Fig. 9.3 Multiple Piconets in Bluetooth for Health Monitoring

The existing ad hoc networks do not use sophisticated multi-hop routing protocols that are necessary to support health monitoring services. Also, an intelligent power control and management for improved transmission of emergency signals based on the contents of messages must be added. We also assume the presence of multiple routing schemes that can be dynamically chosen for the transmission of signals based on the contents of messages. The existing ad hoc networks do not support such dynamic selection/use of routing schemes. Many of the protocols and enhancements do not exist in the current ad hoc networks. These include reliable transmission of emergency signals by using repeated transmissions combined with acknowledgements. Although, it is possible to introduce some of these enhancements in the existing ad hoc wireless networks, the amount of overhead may increase significantly.

In addition, there are many other issues that may also limit the use of existing ad hoc networks for health monitoring. These are possible crowding of ISM bands by the presence of other wireless LANs, interference from medical and other devices generating signals in ISM bands, and the usable capacity of ISM bands for transmitting a large number of vital signs for many patients frequently. Some of these issues can be somewhat alleviated by careful placement of other wireless networks that are not used for health monitoring. It is also possible to use higher ISM bands or even a dedicated band for health monitoring. The availability of a wider dedicated band will significantly improve both the quality and quantity of monitoring services for patients.

9.4 Monitoring Protocols

The vital signs of patients under wireless health monitoring must be obtained, amplified, and converted to digital signals before getting transmitted over ad hoc wireless networks. There are multiple ways to obtain vital signs non-invasively such as multiple sensors on a patient body, specialized bands and wearable monitors, smart shirts, and watch-type wearable devices. It is envisioned that a patient is likely to have diversity of non-invasive and wearable devices. The proposed configuration for health monitoring device is shown in Figure 9.4, where vital signs are acquired as analog signals and processed, followed by conversion to digital signals. Then the vitals signs can be stored, displayed and transmitted over ad hoc wireless networks to healthcare professionals for suitable actions on healthcare delivery.

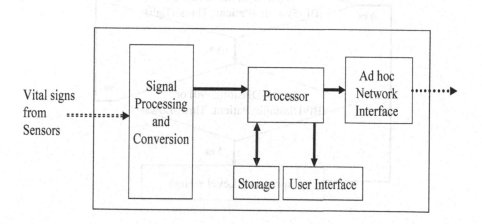

Fig. 9.4 Configuration of Health Monitoring Device

A protocol is also needed in determining when and how vital signs will be measured, checked and coded for transmission. A multi-thresholds based protocols for detecting emergency and abnormal events can be utilized, where one or more events are generated based on levels and patterns of current vital signs. The health monitoring device receives patient's medical information, including personalized thresholds and frequency of monitoring for individual vital signs. This will lead to personalized monitoring for emergency events. For simple health monitoring devices, this information could be obtained from the patient database, while more sophisticated health monitoring devices could store it locally. Once the vital signs are acquired, threshold and pattern-based processing is done to determine the level of emergency and a suitable action is taken, such as generation of a transmission event with a certain priority. A simple example is shown in Figure 9.5 for decision-making for emergencies using blood pressure.

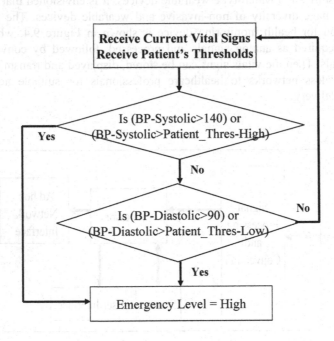

Fig. 9.5 Decision Making for Emergencies using Patient's BP

9.5 Routing in Ad Hoc Networks

Ad hoc networks offer flexibility and can be formed or removed easily. In ad hoc networks, there is no centralized or fixed infrastructure (base stations), unlike in infrastructure-oriented wireless networks. Although ad hoc networks offer almost unrestricted mobility, but the routing become very complex due to the lack of centralized infrastructure. In ad hoc networks, each device is capable of acting as a router. The end-to-end communications between two devices is possible only by the co-operation of devices. This includes routing of messages, which experiences difficulty due to user mobility, transmitted power budget, and multiple problems related to the wireless channels. Due to user mobility, many routes become unusable, resulting in discovery of new routes or rerouting of old routes (Figure 9.6). Devices with more battery power and functionality can act as group leader and in some cases can also connect with the rest of the world using network interface to other wireless networks (such as satellites).

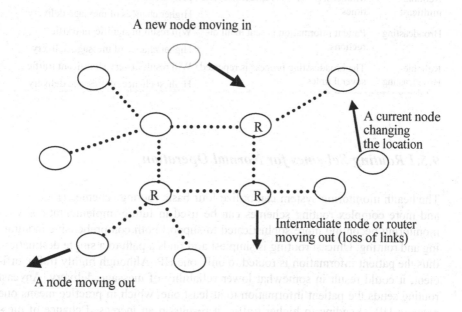

Fig. 9.6 Some Problems in Ad Hoc Networks

The routers agree to use a routing scheme, such as unicast, where a path to the desired destination is discovered and each router on that path stores the next-hop (who is the next router) information in a table. The table gets updated as necessary with changes in the path or due to the mobility of one or more routers.

There are several different types of routing schemes that can be used in ad hoc wireless networks for health monitoring. Table 9.1 shows many of these routing schemes.

Table 9.1 Various Routing Schemes for Ad Hoc Networks

Routing Scheme	Description	Comment
Regular routing (unicast)	Patient information is routed to one and only one health care personnel	Most efficient routing
		Lower chances of message delivery
Anycast routing	Patient information is routed to multiple healthcare personnel	Higher traffic
		Increased chances of message delivery
Multicast routing	Patient information is multicast to multiple healthcare personnel	Requires creation of multicast tree or structure (so some delays)
		Efficient routing
		Increased chances of message delivery
Reliable-multicast	Multicast process is repeated several times	Increased traffic
		Higher chances of message delivery
Broadcasting	Patient information is sent in all directions	Will result in significant traffic
		Higher chance of message delivery
Reliable-Broadcasting	The broadcasting process is repeated several times	Will result in very significant traffic
		Highest chance of message delivery

9.5.1 Routing Schemes for Normal Operation

The health monitoring system can utilize four basic routing schemes (Figure 9.7), and more complex routing schemes can be used in future implementations with monitoring becoming more sophisticated to support both comprehensive monitoring and routing. Unicast routing is simplest and finds a path to a single destination, thus the patient information is routed to only one HP. Although highly traffic efficient, it could result in somewhat lower reliability of message delivery. Anycast routing sends the patient information to at least one, which in practice means one or more HPs. Leading to higher traffic, it results in an increased chance of message delivery. Multicast routing involve transmission to a certain sub-set of healthcare professionals using a multicast tree (so some delays), but the reliability is significantly enhanced. Broadcast routing, where patient information is sent in all directions to all HPs, will lead to the highest reliability of message delivery, but the resulting network traffic can be excessive. More details of unicast, Anycast, multicast and broadcast are shown in Figures 9.8-9.11, respectively.

In addition, more persistent versions of routing can be used such as reliable multicast and reliable broadcast, which involve repeated transmission of information on multiple paths (some old and some newly discovered) in wireless ad hoc networks. These can lead to significantly higher reliability, thus becoming more suitable for emergency messages. The implementation supports the switching among routing schemes to support a range of required performance for messages of different levels of emergencies.

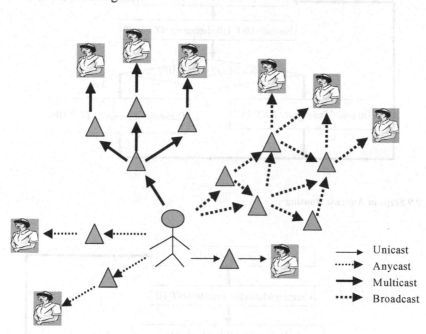

Fig. 9.7 Four Common Routing Schemes for Ad Hoc Networks

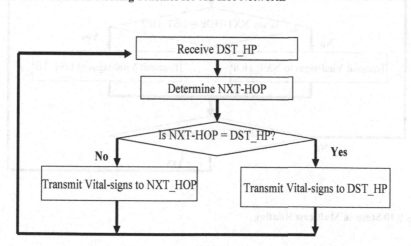

Fig. 9.8 Steps in Unicast Routing

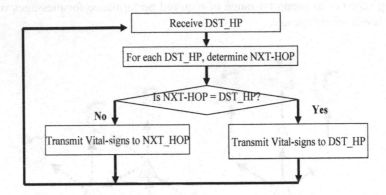

Fig. 9.9 Steps in Anycast Routing

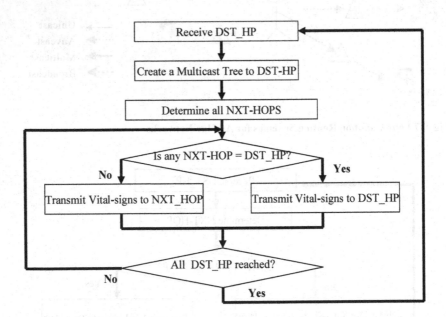

Fig. 9.10 Steps in Multicast Routing

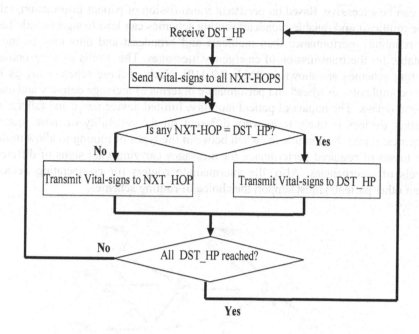

Fig. 9.11 Steps in Broadcast Routing

9.5.2 Routing For Emergencies

The support for emergency messages in health monitoring requires very high reliability of message delivery, low delays and minimal message corruption. For an ad hoc wireless network, emergency messages can be transmitted to healthcare professionals using two different routing schemes (Figure 9.12). The routing schemes differ in how messages are routed to a destination, thus affecting the reliability of message delivery and network traffic, which also affects the end-to-end delay, a critical factor in the transmission of emergency messages in wireless health monitoring.

In addition to multicast and broadcast routing, two more routing schemes are proposed here for emergency messages. These include reliable multicast and reliable broadcast [10]. In multicast routing, patient information is sent to multiple, not all, healthcare professionals. This requires creation of multicast tree or structure (so some delays), but the reliability of message delivery is significantly enhanced. Broadcast routing, where patient information is sent in all directions to all nodes, will lead to the best reliability of message delivery, but the resulting network traffic can be excessive. Based on persistent transmission of patient information, reliable multicast and reliable broadcast routing schemes can lead to significantly better reliability performance than multicast and broadcast and thus may be more suitable for the transmission of emergency messages. The details of the proposed routing schemes are shown in Table 9.2 [10]. Each of these schemes brings its own complexity, overhead and performance in terms of message delivery and end-to-end delays. The impact of patient mobility, limited device range and failures of routing devices is likely to be very different on the reliability of these routing schemes. It may be possible to switch between the types of routing to allow multiple levels of required performance for messages carrying vital-signs of different levels of emergencies. Also, the intermediate routers (or co-operating devices from other patients) must support the choice of routing schemes.

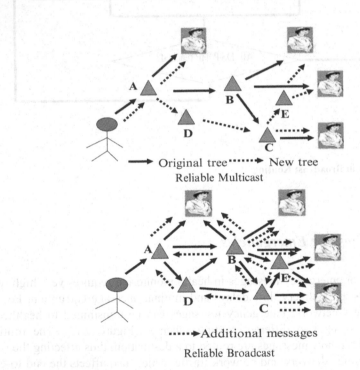

Fig. 9.12 Reliable Multicast and Reliable Broadcast Routing

Table 9.2 Routing Schemes for Health Monitoring

Routing	Computations
Multicast	**Source device**
Routing	{Receive DST_HP (*List of healthcare professionals*)

Create MCAST_TREE (*Form a multicast tree to healthcare professionals*)

Determine ALL_NXT_HOPS (*Find all next hop devices on the multicast tree*)

Send VTL_SGNS to ALL_NXT_HOPS}

Intermediate device

{Determine ALL_NXT_HOPS

If any NXT_HOP = DST_HP (*If any next hop is one of the destinations, routing is completed*)

      Send VTL_SGNS to DST_HP

Else

      Send VTL_SGNS to ALL_NXT_HOPS (*Send vital signs to all the next hops on the multicast tree*)}

Broadcast routing **Source device**

{Receive DST_HP (*List of healthcare professionals*)

Send VTL_SGNS to ALL_NXT_HOPS}

Intermediate device

{Determine ALL_NXT_HOPS

(*Except the one where packet came from*)

Send VTL_SGNS to ALL_NXT_HOPS

(*Send vital signs to all the next hops*)}

Reliable multicast **Source device**

{Receive DST_HP (*List of healthcare professionals*)

Generate DEVICE_LST (*Include all devices*)

For I=1 to Max

Create MCAST_TREE [I] using DEVICE_LST(*Form Ith multicast tree to healthcare professionals*)

Determine ALL_NXT_HOPS (*Find all next hop devices on the multicast tree*)

Send VTL_SGNS to ALL_NXT_HOPS

Update DEVICE_LST (*Remove un-cooperative devices*)}

Intermediate device

{Determine ALL_NXT_HOPS

If any NXT_HOP = DST_HP (*If any next hop is one of the destinations, routing is completed*)

      Send VTL_SGNS to DST_HP

Else

      Send VTL_SGNS to ALL_NXT_HOPS (*Send vital signs to all the next hops on the multicast tree*)}

Reliable broadcast **Source device**

```
{Receive DST_HP (*List of healthcare professionals*)
Send VTL_SGNS to ALL_NXT_HOPS}
Intermediate device
For I=1 to Max
{Determine ALL_NXT_HOPS
(*Include the one where packet came from*)
Send VTL_SGNS to ALL_NXT_HOPS
(*Send vital signs to all the next hops*)}
```

9.6 Reliability of Ad Hoc Network Monitoring

One of the most difficult challenges in health monitoring using wireless networks, especially for emergency messages, is the reliability of message delivery. The unpredictable reliability of health monitoring could lead to difficulty in achieving continuous health monitoring and delivery of monitoring signals from a patient to healthcare professionals, and eventually, the delayed medical response to patients could result in injury. To support the reliability and monitoring delay requirements of health monitoring, significant work is necessary in creating wireless network architecture and protocols to support routing and delivery of messages carrying a range of vital signs and healthcare information. In addition to routing schemes such as multicast and broadcast and protocols for messages carrying vital signs, several enhancements can be added to further improve the reliability of message delivery over ad hoc wireless networks. The following enhancements can be considered [1]:
(a) using multiple ad hoc networks
(b) increasing the number of healthcare professionals
(c) using network or middleware protocols for higher reliability
(d) improving power transmission

9.6.1 Use of Multiple Ad Hoc Networks

This could involve using more than one ad hoc network for messages requiring very reliable transmission. In some ways, this is conceptually similar to multi-path routing such as multicast or broadcast, but access to multiple networks may allow overcoming the unusual situations such as failure of routers/devices. From the power transmission point of view, this is not the best strategy, but is suited for highly reliable transmissions. Also, for enhanced reliability of message delivery, ad hoc networks can be proactively formed even with an increased processing and storage for maintaining, updating and creating ad hoc networks.

9.6.2 Increasing the Number of HP and Devices

By increasing the number of healthcare professionals with devices, the network can increase the chance that one of them will receive the message. This assumes that emergency messages can be delivered to any or more than one healthcare professionals. In cases of fixed assignment of a certain healthcare professional to the monitored patient, this will not work. Increasing the number of devices (fixed or mobile) that can be used for routing will increase the richness of network connectivity and a higher chance of message delivery. Some of these are shown in Figure 9.13.

9.6.3 Design of Network or Middleware Protocols

The protocols could involve more persistent transmission of vital signs with higher reliability requirements, use of acknowledgements, and transmission of differential signals to reduce the power requirements.

9.6.4 Improved Power Management

In ad hoc networks, the amount of power transmitted will affect both the ability of a health monitoring device to transmit emergency messages and the end-to-end delivery of these messages. In general, an increased power transmission will improve the chances of finding co-operating devices or a healthcare professional. But on the other side, monitoring devices should conserve power to allow their continued operation. The power management could include the transmission of minimal power to reach to the next co-operating device, resulting in a higher level of power conservation and could also lead to an increased level of participation from devices with limited power budget. These enhancements can be supported by informing simple health monitoring devices the level of power necessary to reach to the next hop and more complex devices to keep track of required power levels from prior transmissions and/or signals from neighboring hops. Addition enhancements for better power management include (a) minimizing the frequency and the number of vital signs that must be transmitted and (b) special coding and compression of vital signs, including differential ones, to reduce the number of bits that must be transmitted by the health monitoring device. The monitoring devices can also go to sleep to conserve their power when not in use.

More work is needed in deriving how to keep device and network protocols simplest and minimal overhead (to conserve battery) by minimizing the amount of information transmitted from patient's device. This could include use of other devices to proxy for the patient's device and send information thus reducing the amount of information from the patient's device. On one hand, things should be simple, but not too inefficient as monitoring devices need conserve power to help owners/patients.

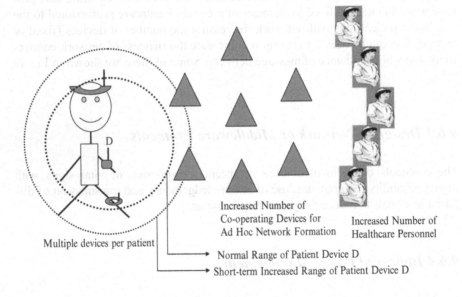

Multiple devices per patient

Increased Number of Co-operating Devices for Ad Hoc Network Formation

Increased Number of Healthcare Personnel

→ Normal Range of Patient Device D

→ Short-term Increased Range of Patient Device D

Fig. 9.13 Several Different Ways to Improve Reliability of Monitoring

9.7 Future

The role played by ad hoc networks is likely to be supplemental, extending the coverage to isolated and remote areas and providing back-up coverage to infrastructure-oriented wireless networks. In practice, the end-to-end health monitoring network would be a combination of ad hoc and infrastructure-oriented wireless networks. The examples could include Bluetooth and cellular/3G network, Bluetooth and 802.11 wireless LAN, ad hoc network implementation and cellular/3G network. Ad hoc wireless networks based monitoring could be suitable for emergencies and for cases where a few patients need to be monitored for longer terms.

Questions:

1. How would monitoring devices know when and how to form ad hoc networks?
2. Why would hybrid configuration most likely to be used in practice for WHM?
3. Identify the major challenges in ad hoc networks for WHM. Discuss one of these in more details.
4. Compare different schemes for routing patient information through ad hoc wireless networks.
5. Compare schemes for routing of emergency messages.
6. In practice, the devices are more likely to be clustered and not uniformly distributed. Make some comments on routing through clusters.
7. Discuss how sleep cycles may affect the reliability of WHM.
8. Make a business case for using ad hoc networks for WHM. The proposal about must show how the benefits, brought by the reliability, speed, and correctness, can outweigh the efficiency in terms of cost savings and quality of services.
9. Think of ways how routing tables can be updated in ad hoc networks.

References
[1] Varshney U (2004) Using wireless networks for enhanced monitoring of patients. In Proc. Americas Conference on Information Systems, August
[2] Varshney U (2003) Pervasive healthcare. IEEE Computer, 36(12):138-140, December
[3] Varshney U, Sneha S (2006) Patient monitoring using ad hoc wireless networks: reliability and power management. IEEE Communications Magazine, 44(4): 49-55, April
[4] Lorincz K, et. al (2004) Sensor networks for emergency response: challenges and opportunities. IEEE Pervasive Computing, 3(4): 16-23, Oct-Dec.
[5] Lee D, Lee Y, Chung W, and Myllyla R (2006) Vital sign monitoring system with life emergency event detection using wireless sensor network. In Proc. IEEE Conference on Sensors, 518-521
[6] Radenkovic M, Wietrzyk B (2006) Mobile ad hoc networking approach to detecting and querying events related to farm animals. In Proc. Int. conference on Networking and Services (ICNS '06), 109
[7] Hongliang R, Meng M (2006) Understanding the mobility model of wireless body sensor networks. In Proc. IEEE International Conference on Information Acquisition, 306-310
[8] Parkka J, Van Gils M, Tuomisto T, Lappalainen R, Korhonen I (2000), A wireless wellness monitor for personal weight management. In Proc. 22nd Annu. Int. Conf. IEEE Eng. Med. Biol. Soc, 83-88
[9] Lamprinos I, Prentza A, Sakke E, Koutsouris (2004) A low power medium access control protocol for wireless medical sensor networks. In Proc. 26th IEEE EMBS Annual International Conference, 2129-2132
[10] Varshney U (2008) A framework for supporting emergency messages in wireless patient monitoring. Decision Support Systems, 45(4): 981-996, November

Chapter 10 Using Incentives in Wireless Health Monitoring

Abstract With an increasing healthcare cost and a growing population of seniors and disabled worldwide, there is a need to provide quality healthcare services using limited financial and human resources. Health monitoring of patients using wireless LANs and cellular networks has begun in indoor and outdoor environments. Recently, health monitoring using ad hoc wireless networks, formed among devices when the coverage of infrastructure-oriented wireless networks is not available, has been proposed. Although innovative, such ad hoc networks primarily rely on the co-operation of devices and any lack of co-operation negatively affects the delivery of messages carrying patients' vital signs. We discuss how reliable wireless health monitoring can be achieved using ad hoc networks, ways to obtain the cooperation of routing devices, and an incentive-based mechanism to improve wireless health monitoring. The design of protocols is also presented for decision making in incentive-driven environment.

10.1 Introduction

There has been some work in health monitoring using computing devices and networks. This includes identification of challenges associated with comprehensive patient monitoring [1]. For obtaining vital-signs of patients on continuous or on-demand basis, several wearable and portable monitoring devices using a variety of sensors have become possible including Smart Shirt [3], commercially available LifeShirt [4], and networked monitoring devices [5]. The work on networked patient monitoring includes specifying requirements for generating alerts in patient monitoring [6], wireless application protocol (WAP)-based patient monitoring [7], sensors-based stress monitoring [8], and, wireless patient monitoring [9].

One of the most difficult challenges in health monitoring using wireless networks is the reliability of message delivery. The quality of health monitoring is also affected by the end-to-end monitoring delays, the frequency of monitoring, and the number of patients that need to be monitored.

Many hospitals and nursing homes are using infrastructure-oriented wireless networks, such as IEEE 802.11 wireless LANs and cellular systems [1, 5]. The fixed infrastructure supports some mobility of patients by allowing their devices to access one of several base stations (cellular networks) or access points (wireless LANs). To supplement the coverage of infrastructure-oriented wireless networks,

U. Varshney, *Pervasive Healthcare Computing: EMR/EHR, Wireless and Health Monitoring*, 211
DOI: 10.1007/978-1-4419-0215-3_10,
© Springer Science + Business Media, LLC 2009

several health monitoring devices can form an ad hoc network for transmission of monitoring messages [9]. Although a very innovative solution to provide health monitoring, the use of ad hoc wireless networks assumes that all routers are co-operative, functioning properly, and trust-worthy. In real-life, some routers, especially those owned by different entities, will not be co-operative, some will experience failures, and some will not be trust-worthy for healthcare information. In general, the non-cooperation could occur due to the following reasons. Some users may not want their devices to act as routers, so could decide to shut-off when they feel that the devices will not be needed to transmit their own monitoring signals anytime soon. Some devices may be programmed to save energy, thus become unwilling to route packets of others. These could include devices that are already in sleep cycle, thus not able to receive and route packets or about to go to sleep and thus not able to route packets. Although failures are not common, some devices may experience failures related to hardware, batteries, and network access over a certain time. Also routing devices owned by different entities may not co-operate in routing of patient messages or may exhibit intermittent co-operation. This could be part of their administrative policy as part of security precautions to not become a carrier of hackers. The rest of the problems could be attributed to router misbehavior due to several known and unknown reasons.

A possible scenario is shown in Figure 10.1, where both inter- and intra-body area networks (BAN) may be implemented as ad hoc wireless networks. In general, devices in the same intra-body area network serving the same patient are likely to co-operate for routing. More likely, the problem could exist in intra-body area network. Here, routers have several problems. This includes D who is non co-operative, B who is experiencing failure, and F who is out of range. While making the routing of packets difficult, these problems are not easy to solve. In case of routing involving D2, C, and D, a message will not be delivered to healthcare professional (HP3). The same is true for D2, D1 and F. Fortunately, the message will reach to HP1 when D2, D1, G, I or H are involved. The message will reach HP2 via D2, C, and E. However, if C and G were not co-operative, the message would not reach to any of the four healthcare professionals, showing the extreme impact of router non-cooperation on wireless health monitoring. In this chapter, we discuss how incentives can be used to obtain co-operation from routers and thus improve the reliability of wireless health monitoring. This cannot be applied to other problems (Figure 10.1) of router failure, but the router F, who is out of range, could increase the level of transmitted power to route the message for earning incentives.

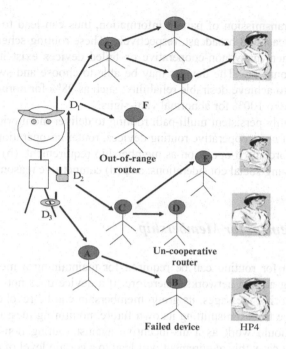

Fig. 10.1 Non Co-operative Routers

10.2 Overcoming the Non-cooperation of Routers

In general, there are several different techniques to overcome potential routing problems due to non-cooperative and/or failed routers: (a) persistent transmission involving non-cooperating devices, which may eventually transmit at reduced power level if the distance reduces, (b) use of persistent multi-path routing schemes such as reliable multicast and reliable broadcast, and, (c) exclude non-cooperative devices from the routes as in multicast tree.

These techniques can be utilized in the routing schemes, for the ad hoc network based health monitoring system, including multicast, reliable multicast, broadcast, and reliable broadcast. In multicast routing, the patient information is sent to multiple, but not all, healthcare professionals. This requires creation of multicast tree or a structure with increased control traffic and processing, but the reliability of delivery can be enhanced by excluding non-cooperating devices from the chosen routes. Broadcast routing, where patient information is sent in all directions to all nodes, will lead to higher reliability of message delivery, but at excessive network traffic. Compared to multicast, broadcast routing can generally handle a higher level of non-cooperation. Reliable multicast and Reliable broadcast schemes utilize a persistent transmission of patient information, thus can lead to higher reliability than multicast and broadcast, respectively. These routing schemes may be more suitable when many non-cooperative or failed devices exist in the health monitoring environment. The devices may be able to choose and switch among routing schemes to achieve desirable reliability, such as 98% for normal-range vital signs and close to 100% for abnormal vital-signs.

In addition to highly persistent multi-path routing to deliver monitoring messages in the presence of non-cooperative routing devices, router co-operation can be obtained by (a) enforcing co-operation as membership requirement, (b) offering incentives, (c) utilizing social considerations, and (d) competitive reasons.

10.2.1 Requirement for Membership

The co-operation for routing can be required for maintaining a membership in health monitoring ad hoc networks. Therefore, if a device does not route certain number of monitoring messages, its group membership can be revoked. This will prevent the device from transmitting its own future monitoring messages over the network. This should work as a dis-incentive against routing non-cooperation. Even in the worst case, this requirement will lead to a certain level of co-operation from routing devices. In practice, routing behavior for every device will be monitored by other devices. This "peer review" will result in some storage and processing overhead based on the network traffic and the number of routing devices.

10.2.2 Incentives

To encourage co-operation, a range of incentives from payments to future higher priority for their messages can be offered. The routing devices can make a decision whether to co-operate or not based on offered incentives, already earned incentives, and the energy cost of routing. The payments for routing co-operation could include processing and networking resources, which can be used later for transmission of their own packets [10]. The router co-operation can also be attempted by using priority-based forwarding, where messages from a device are forwarded based on its own history of co-operation. Also, higher incentives for routing an emergency message could encourage, or even lead to some competition among, routers for such messages. For devices recently joining an ad hoc network and the ones coming out of failures, a "default" priority can assigned (medium or high) based on their future co-operation in routing. Also, a forced resetting (lowering) of priority may be used as a dis-incentive against devices trying to claim "failed" status.

10.2.3 Social Considerations

In some cases, enforcing membership rules will be difficult if multiple diverse domains are involved. Also, the overhead cost of peer review of routing behavior could become prohibitive. The incentive-based protocols may be complex or in some cases not attractive enough for obtaining the co-operation from routing devices. In such cases, other factors such as social consideration can be utilized. These may include the natural willingness to help your friends, inclination to charitable behavior, and even use of reputation. An example would be a patient's device programmed to route messages of his/her friends, which could be extended to include a community of people such as everyone in a nursing home. Also, some patients may be more willing to have their devices act as routers for forwarding of messages as an act of charity. This charity could be rewarded by adding a higher status on these devices, which will enable them to receive future routing support for their own messages.

The use of reputation can also be used in routing [11] and protocols for detecting selfish nodes can also be considered [12]. In reputation-based systems [11], nodes detect selfish nodes by using second-hand information and work on isolating these nodes from the network. The potential damage caused by incorrect information must be considered in such system where a group of devices could isolate one or more co-operative nodes. For health monitoring, the impact of such isolation due to faulty information can be very significant, especially if it affects future emergency messages or alerts. The use of acknowledgements in avoiding routes involving selfish nodes is proposed in [12], where a higher level protocol is added on the top of a routing scheme to detect selfish nodes.

10.2.4 Competitive Angle

In cases, where multiple paths could exist for routing a message, such as those in some ad hoc networks and in mesh networks, a node could become aware that there are some competing nodes which could also be offered the same incentives to get their routing co-operation. Now as the node knows that another node on the competing path may get these incentives, it could somehow include this in the decision making. Therefore, it is not just incentive but the threat of incentives going to a competitor, who could use this to dictate terms in the future to get more control over routing and better quality of service for its own packets. The level of earned incentives may also be used in selecting which devices can act as network monitors or sleep coordinators, who may influence the network even more.

One way to implement competitive routing is to allow routers to bid their prices of routing. This information can be made known to other devices along with their current locations. This will help in a source device knowing the level of incentives it has to offer, the number of routers willing to route its message, and the current location of potential routers.

We have so far presented several different ways to obtain routing co-operation. To put all of these in perspective, these techniques are compared in Table 10.1.

Table 10.1. Several different techniques for routing co-operation and message delivery

Technique	Advantage	Limitation	Comment
Multi-path routing (highly persistent)	Higher reliability of delivery	Excessive traffic	Poor scalability due to traffic and power consumption
Membership requirements	Certain level of co-operation achievable	Monitoring of nodes' routing behavior	Limit on how much co-operation is achieved
Incentives	Encourages nodes to co-operate	Processing and storage overhead	Will work if nodes exhibit "rational" behavior
Social consideration	Use of social constructs in support for routing	Evaluating the effectiveness	May not work in all conditions
Competitive angle	Can motivate a router to provide co-operation	Difficulty in decision making	Will work only if competition for routing exists

10.3 Incentives for Co-operation of Devices

As discussed in section 10.2, there are several ways to achieve co-operation from routers. In this section, we focus on using incentives for obtaining router co-operation. The impact of incentives is likely to vary significantly from one scenario to another. For example, when all nodes are administered by a single entity, the router co-operation could be easily obtained. However, when different users and administrative entities may have somewhat conflicting goals, the co-operation may not be easy. But then, offering incentives to obtain router co-operation could become very useful. Next, we discuss how incentives, called Vital-credits [10], can be used to achieve co-operation from routing devices.

To obtain the co-operation for routing, routing devices will be offered per-message Vital-credits based on (a) the priority level of message, (b) the current network load, and (c) the criticality of the router. The criticality can be derived based on the device position and the current routing scheme. The criticality would be lower in cases of multi-path routing or for topologies where an alternate node for routing can be easily found. The criticality is also a dynamic factor and its value can change easily based on the mobility, availability and/or failure of other nodes. If suddenly several other nodes become available for routing, the criticality of a node will go down.

The routing devices can decide whether to co-operate or not based on (a) the offered incentives, (b) the current level of stored or already earned incentives, and (c) their current power levels. This process is shown in Figure 10.2, where an Incentive Estimator, running at source device, derives Vital-credits for the current message. The co-operation protocol, running on individual routing devices, is then used to decide whether to co-operate or not. For implementation purposes, these decisions functions could be supported by some devices which can then communicate the decisions to the nodes involved.

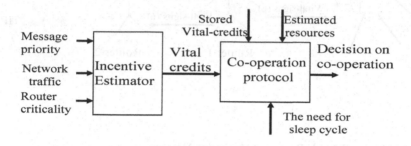

Fig. 10.2 Incentive Generation and Decision Making

Assuming rational behavior, a device is more likely to co-operate if its stored Vital-credits are smaller and the offered Vitals-credits are proportionately higher. Also, a device with large value of stored Vital-credits is unlikely to co-operate even if the offered incentives were high. Factors such as a recent sleep cycle or the need to go through another sleep cycle soon, along with current power levels of devices can also influence the outcome. The routing devices need to keep track of routing credits, which can be done by Credit Manager. An example of end-to-end routing of a message with all the steps is shown in Figure 10.3.

That devices will use stored and offered Vital-credits in making a decision whether to co-operate or not seems to be a reasonable model of their behavior, however, more work is necessary to include devices with unpredictable or irrational behavior in decision making and/or random failures. Also, Nash Equilibrium, when all devices generate their best decisions by also considering decisions of others, can be studied. The maximum reliability for the whole network can also be derived and the scenarios when it can be achieved can also be studied.

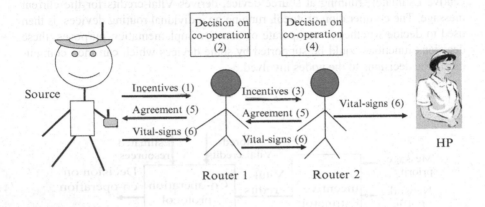

Fig. 10.3 Various Steps in Routing of Monitoring Messages

10.4 Steps in Obtaining Co-operation

The following steps will be used in obtaining co-operation from routing devices. This includes generation of health monitoring messages, finding the next-hop, generation of vital-credits, offering of vital-credits, decision on co-operation, and use of vital-credits for sleep cycle.

10.4.1 Generation of Health Monitoring Messages

The source device, such as a body-sensing wearable computer, monitors the vital signs and parameters of its patient. Based on a threshold event, such as certain time or levels of vital signs exceeding "individualized" thresholds, it generates health monitoring information. The information is then digitized and one or more packets are prepared. Depending on the vital signs, the level of emergency can also be indicated.

10.4.2 Finding the Next-hop

The source device determines the next-hop or it may be already known in a pre-established ad hoc network using a certain routing schemes. In some cases, where the next-hop node has gone to sleep or has a history of non-cooperation, a different next-hop node should be tried.

10.4.3 Generation of Vital-credits

Vital-credits are calculated based on the message priority, network traffic, and criticality of next-hop node. Any potential saving in network traffic can also be used in determining Vital-credits. More complex algorithms can also be used and the derivation of vital-credits could be assisted by more powerful devices.

10.4.4 Offering of Vital-credits

The source device offers Vital-credits to the next-hop node and if an agreement is reached, the source device transmits vital-signs and parameters (Figure 10.4).

10.4.5 Decision on Co-operation

Each device that is offered Vital-credits will decide based on (a) stored Vital-credits, (b) offered Vital-credits, and (c) resources available and needed for the routing (Figure 10.5). If the device agrees to co-operate, the Vital-credits are added to the router (and deducted from the source device).

For multi-hop routing, there are two possibilities: (1) the source device agrees to pay Vital-credits to all co-operative devices on the way to a healthcare professional with or without prior negotiation or (2) the source device offers a fixed number of Vital-credits for the delivery of the message to a healthcare professional. For the first case, the source device may be penalized for any inefficiency in routing, and, there may be an uncertainty on the eventual cost of message delivery. The per-hop incentives will also act as a dis-incentive against multi-path routing such as multicast or broadcast. For the second case, the source device will have to deal with uncertainty on message delivery. Also, for a routing device, the amount of actual Vital-credits will be based on the offered Vital-credits by the source device and the number of devices needed to deliver the message. In both cases, the next-hop device will decide on how much incentive to offer to second-hop device. If the second-hop device does not co-operate, the first-hop device may not be able to keep all Vital-credits. In case of predetermined values of Vital-credits, the source device may opt to choose a certain path, or part of it, to minimize the amount of Vital-credits it needs to spend for the delivery of the message.

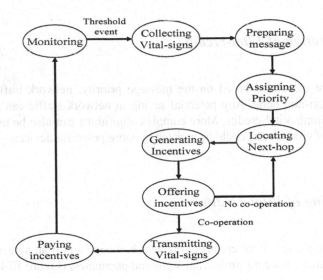

Fig. 10.4 State Diagram for Monitoring Devices

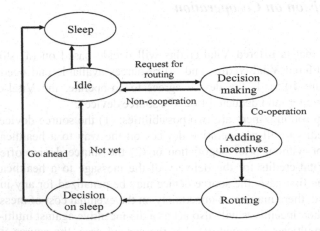

Fig. 10.5 State Diagram for Routing Devices

From a 3-layer view (application, middleware and wireless layers), the health monitoring application runs at the application layer and generates monitoring messages. The search for the next hop is conducted by middleware with the help of wireless network layer. The incentive generation and management are mostly middleware functions, while the routing and power management functions are in the wireless network layer. The layers within a device co-operate with one another and an inter-layer communication is utilized for obtaining co-operation for routing of messages. More work can be done in studying non-cooperation at different layers and among layers.

10.4.6 Use of Vital-credits for Sleep-Cycle

For power conservation purposes, routing devices can apply to go to sleep, if they have sufficient stored credits that are more than needed for their own transmission of packets in the near future. We propose that Vital-credits could be spent by devices to acquire the permission for sleep-cycle. Some devices with more computing and storage functionalities will be assigned the role of sleep coordinators, which will determine whether and when a device can go to sleep for how long, possibly by considering criticality and device density, or the number of devices in a certain area. Sleep-coordinators may also route messages, which would have been processed by the devices currently under sleep, and could earn Vital-credits.
The devices with the most Vital-credits can also be prioritized for sleep-cycle. This will allow Vital-credits to be used as incentives both for routing as well as energy conservation by using sleep-cycles. Also, the devices that have spent Vital-credits for a recent sleep-cycle are more likely to co-operate for packet routing to reach to the same level of Vital-credits as before. It is in the best interest of a device or node to have as much stored credits as possible, subject to its power limitation, for supporting higher reliability for its own messages in the future.

10.5 Protocols and Operations

10.5.1 Traffic Estimation

The network traffic level needs to be estimated and then using message priority, the level of offered incentives can be measured. The traffic could depend on the number of patients that are being monitored, the frequency of monitoring, the number of packets per monitored event, and the current routing scheme. For some simple cases, traffic can be measured using the queue-lengths at different routing devices.

10.5.2 Incentive Estimation

Based on the current network traffic, the priority of the health monitoring message, and the criticality of the device acting as a router, broad incentives can be estimated [10] in terms of Vital-credits as follows

$$I = NT^A \times MP^B \times DC^C \tag{1}$$

Where NT is the current network traffic, MP is the message priority, and DC is the device criticality. The values of A, B, and C can be dynamically chosen to model different environments of wireless health monitoring and/or dynamically changing needs and characteristics of a given monitoring environment. One reason that the equation uses three factors in a multiplicative (and not additive) order is to avoid one factor overwhelming affecting the value of incentives. Certainly, many more different ways of generating incentives can be devised and compared for highest effectiveness in the future. The future work may also have to address incentive re-negotiation if the source device is not able to get co-operation from other routers. Such renegotiations are likely to involve an increased level of incentives, especially for higher level of emergency messages.

10.5.3 Characterization of Devices

The devices need to make a decision whether to route a message or not. The devices can use simple comparisons involving offered Vital-credits, current levels of stored Vital-credits, and their power levels. The comparisons could involve the absolute values of offered and stored Vital-credits, or simply the normalized values. Based on this a device is more likely to co-operate if its stored Vital-credits are less and the offered Vitals-credits are proportionately higher. On the other side, a device with large value of stored Vital-credits is unlikely to co-operate even if the offered incentives were high. Many factors such as the recent sleep cycle or the need to go through a sleep cycle, along with power levels of devices can influence the outcome of incentive-based co-operation. The routing credits can also be used to pay for sleep cycles or for future rejections of routing (there can be negative routing credits for refusing to route packets). It is assumed that devices will use a combination of stored and offered Vital-credits in making a decision whether to co-operate or not. While this seems to be a reasonable model of their behavior, more work should be done towards including a diverse set of devices where some devices may show much more unpredictable behavior in decision making and/or random failures.

10.6 The Decision Making Protocols

The devices can utilize offered Vital-credits, current stored Vital-credits, and their power levels in the decision making on whether to route a health monitoring message or not. The routing devices need to keep track of routing credits (exact or approximate). This is done by Credit Manager, which also plays a role in managing credits and estimation of incentives.

To implement decision making, there is a need for protocols that can perform decisions on whether to co-operate or not based on several factors. Although many different protocols can be designed to support such decisions, we present two protocols based on the level of complexity and accuracy in decision-making for co-operation [10]. These protocols are named Exact Value Protocol (EVP) and Discrete Value Protocol (DVP). The protocols are compared in Table 10.2.

Table 10.2. Comparison of EVP and DVP

Protocol	Designed for	Advantage	Limitation
EVP	More powerful devices	More accurate decision making	More complex processing required
DVP	Less powerful devices	Simplified processing	The decision-making relies on approximation

Exact Value Protocol (EVP) is designed for more complex health monitoring and routing devices and larger ad hoc networks, served by potentially multiple entities. By keeping all parameters and computations at exact values, it will result in an accurate decision making. Likely to have more overhead of computation and storage, this protocol is more suited to monitoring devices with complex functionalities. The health monitoring devices running EVP are likely to be more powerful and have functionality for power conservation. As shown in Figure 10.6, the decision-making on cooperation involves checking accurate values of incentives offered, stored incentives, power required and available, and the need to initiate a sleep cycle soon. The values of A and B can be chosen based on desired thresholds. If the values are kept constant, then each subsequent request for routing is subjected to a higher value of vital-credits and a lower value of power required. To avoid this or to keep the same bar for all routing request, the value of A can be reduced in the same proportion as the increase in stored (earned but not spent) credits and also the value of B is increased in the same proportion as the decrease in power available. The value of T, or the time before the device can go to sleep, can be adjusted to reflect the need to go to sleep sooner for power conservation or any delayed sleep due to changes in the sleep priority assigned by some device acting as sleep coordinators.

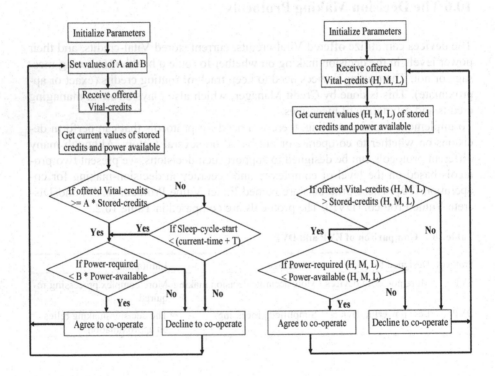

Fig. 10.6 Steps for EVP and DVP

DVP is for simpler health monitoring and routing devices and processes stored incentives and other parameters in some discrete states such as "High", "Medium", and "Low". This will involve using these values for both offered and stored Vital-credits. The network traffic and device criticality will also be represented by a limited number of states. The quantization of a large number of potential values into a few states will simplify computations and resulting overhead but will add some approximation errors in decision making. This is also suited for smaller ad hoc networks and simpler health monitoring devices. As shown in Figure 10.6, the decision-making on cooperation involves checking values of incentives offered, stored incentives, and power required and available. Unlike EVP, DVP does not support sleep cycle for power conservation as health monitoring devices running DVP are unlikely to have the functionality required to create, manage, and execute sleep-cycles for power conservation.

We expect that for smaller values of incentives at low network loads, the performance of EVP and DVP may not differ much. However, EVP is likely to outperform DVP as more accurate decision on co-operation can be made. In general, for both EVP and DVP in ad hoc networks, the reliability of health monitoring will improve with the use of Vital-credits.

10.7 Strategies for Nodes

There are many unanswered questions. In this chapter, we have assumed that once given incentives that a node needs, it will behave rationally and co-operate in routing. But can it be shown that rational behavior is always the best strategy? What if semi-rational or irrational strategies may be better suited for some cases? The semi-rational or irrational strategies may be simpler or may not require much processing, thus saving power consumption of nodes. Certainly, more work is needed in deriving and evaluating the best strategy for a node in terms of whether to co-operate or not. Also, additional work is needed to find if the same strategy is best for both ad hoc networks and mesh networks. If not, then how can these two strategies be derived and utilized?

What if a node uses (a) its own strategy using incentives and power levels, (b) a strategy based on its observation of others involving both scenarios of perfect and imperfect information or (c) a combination of (a) and (b) using local and global information. Certainly the evaluation of such work could lead to many interesting insights. There are several ways to model and evaluate different strategies. This could include game theory, where Nash Equilibrium could occur if each node comes up with its best strategy by also considering the strategy or decision of others. More work is also needed in coming up with the highest possible reliability of message delivery for the whole network and the level of co-operation needed from each node.

For evaluation, the probabilities of different events can be computed and then these strategies can be used to see which one gets the best reliability and power saving for nodes. Some work can also be done in finding out if these strategies ever get to a steady state and how long does it take? If there is no steady state, then lower and upper bound can still be attempted.

10.7.1 Scalability, Predictability and Convergence

The scalability of the incentive-based co-operation in ad hoc networks will depend on the growth of overhead with an increased number of messages, devices, and network size. The scalability is likely to be easier to achieve for DVP due to its reduced overhead than that for EVP, however, the growth of overhead for EVP and DVP must be computed and managed to ensure scalability. The predictability of the incentive-based co-operation will depend on the accuracy of modeling of devices' behavior. We characterize devices to co-operate based on the level of incentives offered and the value of stored (already earned) incentives. As some devices may exhibit more unpredictable behavior and/or experience random failures, modeling should be expanded to include this additional attribute. The convergence to equilibrium for incentive-based cooperation will be based on (a) incentives, (b) modeled behavior, (c) mobility level of devices, (d) power level of devices, and, (e) behavior of vital signs and crossing of thresholds.

One way to manage overhead and thus to improve scalability is to limit the number of packets which are assigned Vital Credits. This means that only emergency packets are assigned Vital-credits and as these are likely to be less frequent than "regular" packets, the overhead of computation and co-operation decision will reduce due to less frequent need to perform these decisions. The other may be to fix the value of vital-credits and then the nodes may use simpler versions of protocols in decision making and thus the overhead is reduced.

10.8 Challenges in the Implementation of Incentives

Several challenges that may arise in the operation of incentive-based co-operation schemes are need for dis-incentives for non-cooperation, potential disagreements over Vital-credits, and, the occurrence of intermittent co-operation.

10.8.1 Dis-incentives for Non-cooperation

To avoid persistent non-cooperation, negative credits can be introduced and enforced if a device does not co-operate for every few high-priority packets. The devices experiencing a failure or spending time in power saving mode without authorization could also be awarded some negative Vital-credits. This would encourage these devices to offer a higher level of co-operation once they are back online. The interaction of dis-incentives with sleep-cycle and device failures needs to be studied in more details. Any potential errors in measuring non-cooperation should also be avoided. More work is also needed to address the possibility of having a node prevented from transmitting its own emergency messages.

10.8.2 Disagreements over Vital-credits

The Vital-credits will be generated, awarded and spent by most devices in the proposed incentive-based cooperation. There may be disagreements among routing devices over the actual amount of Vital-credits due to some differences in protocols (DVP or EVP) used and/or errors in Incentive Managers. To avoid this, periodic checking and settlements of credits and protocol matching can be performed. In some implementations, vital-credits may also have expiration times, to encourage continued co-operation from the nodes as more recent, and not very old, co-operation will reflect in the current value of stored (and not spent) vital-credits.

10.8.3 Dealing with Intermittent Co-operation

Intermittent co-operation could occur due to device problems and failures, sleep cycles, and in some cases also due to the proposed incentive protocols for co-operation especially when a node has earned significant vital-credits. It could affect the end-to-end reliability of message delivery in unpredictable ways. The use of negative Vital-credits can also be instituted to reduce any intermittent co-operation. In practice, dealing with intermittent co-operation is much harder than dealing with simple non-cooperation due to the uncertainty of when a device will co-operate. Certainly more work is needed in designing schemes that can counteract with intermittent co-operation. To start with, first any such intermittent co-operation should be detected and then the exact cause can be found. Then one or more protocols can be designed to handle intermittent co-operation.

10.8.4 Borrowing and Settlement of Vital-credits

To avoid excessive traffic among devices, Vital-credits can be settled on a periodic basis and not per message basis. Also, in some cases, Vital-credits can be borrowed for needed routing of a device's message and can be repaid through the future co-operation of this device for routing of messages from other devices.

10.9 Conclusions and Future Research

Wireless health monitoring using ad hoc networks is a very interesting and important solution for supplementing the coverage of infrastructure-oriented wireless networks. However, such health monitoring heavily relies on the co-operation of devices acting as routers. And the end-to-end delivery of messages carrying vital signs of patients will be negatively affected by any non-cooperation and/or failure of routers. To address this significant problem, several solutions, are presented. More importantly, incentives could be effective in obtaining the co-operation of routers and therefore can lead to significant improvement in the reliability of message delivery. For making such co-operation a reality, the protocols, operation, and related issues of an incentive-based mechanism are also described.

There are many challenges that should be addressed in the future work. These include studying (a) overhead of implementing and utilizing incentive-based schemes, (b) the impact of intermittent and/or selective co-operation, (c) the design of protocols to handle a range of co-operation levels that are time, location and router dependent, and, (d) a comprehensive evaluation under varying device density, intermittently co-operative routers, and diverse failure scenarios of routers. More work is also needed in addressing security vulnerabilities in ad hoc networks, especially when the patient information is transmitted to potentially large number of users such as in broadcast routing.

Questions:

1. Compare several different ways to obtain co-operation from routing devices in ad hoc networks.
2. Discuss if social consideration would be effective in obtaining co-operation from other devices.
3. Will incentives be sufficient for all cases of non-cooperation including failures of devices?
4. Describe the functions of Incentive Manager.
5. What happens if Incentive Manager fails?
6. Design a protocol for more irrational behavior. Note that EVP and DCP are designed for rational behavior.
7. What happens if a device borrows Vital Credits and then it fails or claims a "failed" status?

References
[1] Varshney U (2003) Pervasive healthcare. IEEE Computer, 36(12):138-140, December
[2] Vital Signs: http://www.nlm.nih.gov/medlineplus/ency/article/002341.htm
[3] Smart Shirt: http://www.gtwm.gatech.edu
[4] LifeShirt: http://www.vivometrics.com/site/system.html

[5] Monitoring Devices from WelchAllyn: http://www.monitoring.welchallyn.com/products/wireless/

[6] Kafeza E, Chiu D, Cheung S, Kafeza M (2004) Alerts in mobile healthcare applications: requirements and pilot study. IEEE Trans. Inf. Technol. Biomed, 8(2):173-181, June

[7] Hung K, Zhang Y-T (2003) Implementation of a WAP-based telemedicine system for patient monitoring. IEEE Trans. Inf. Technol. Biomed, 7(2):101-107, June

[8] Jovanov E, et.al (2003) Stress monitoring using a distributed wireless intelligent sensor system. IEEE Engineering in Medicine and Biology Magazine, 22(3):49-55, May-June

[9] Varshney U (2004) Wireless networks for enhanced monitoring of patients. In Proc. Americas Conference on Information Systems (AMCIS), August

[10] Varshney U (2008) Improving wireless health monitoring using incentive-based router cooperation. IEEE Computer, 41(5):56-62, May

[11] Buchegger S, Boudec J-Y (2005) Self-policing mobile ad hoc networks by reputation systems. IEEE Communications Magazine, 43(7): 101-107, July

[12] Balakrishnan K, Deng J, Varshney P (2005) TWOACK: Preventing selfishness in mobile ad hoc networks. In Proc. IEEE Wireless Communications and Networking Conference (WCNC), 2137-2142

Chapter 11: Context-awareness in Healthcare

Abstract Context information in health monitoring can be used to improve the quality of healthcare delivery, utilize limited healthcare and human resources more efficiently, and to better match the healthcare services to the current medical conditions and needs of the patients under health monitoring. This chapter presents why context awareness is desirable for healthcare and how it can be extended to support monitoring of multiple chronic illnesses. More specifically, we address how the context may be generated and utilized in health monitoring. The evolution from context-awareness to health-awareness is also presented along with additional research to address the current problems in context-awareness.

11.1 Introduction

Health monitoring has received some attention from researchers worldwide in the last few years. This has resulted in several prototypes, systems, and applications of health monitoring in a variety of scenarios. Although innovative, such work primarily relies on specialized hardware, software, and communications protocols. Also, with increasing sophistication of monitoring devices, increased reliance on wireless networks, and the need to monitor multiple chronic health conditions, wireless health monitoring is evolving towards the second generation.

There is a need for context information in health monitoring to improve the quality of healthcare delivery, utilize the limited healthcare and human resources more efficiently, and to move towards matching the healthcare services to the current medical conditions and needs of the patients under health monitoring. The context of a patient's current needs can be derived using the patient's medical history, current location and activity, values/rate of changes in the patient's current vital signs, among other pieces of information. Context-aware wireless health monitoring systems can be implemented and utilized to support diverse patients with a range of chronic conditions, using advances in devices, networks, and protocols.

This chapter presents why context awareness is desirable for healthcare, when it may add complexity, uncertainty, difficulty of use, and possible delays in some cases. The work can be extended to support monitoring of multiple chronic illnesses and can be implemented by a range of wireless technologies. Several questions that must be addressed are how to make pervasive healthcare systems and applications context-aware. What is needed and where and how it will be implemented? Which components of pervasive healthcare systems need to have additional functionalities? Would someone use "self supported context awareness" or

U. Varshney, *Pervasive Healthcare Computing: EMR/EHR, Wireless and Health Monitoring*,
DOI: 10.1007/978-1-4419-0215-3_11,
© Springer Science + Business Media, LLC 2009

"infrastructure-based context awareness" for context-awareness? What about user control in different situations involving homecare, assisted living, and nursing home and different type of patients with a range of cognitive and/or physical limitations? What about user preferences for notifications to whom and the type of healthcare services in certain situations?

Also, how to show that context-awareness helps in decision making for healthcare services or wireless health monitoring? Are there cases or scenarios, where context should not be used? Are there healthcare applications it should always be used? How much complexity is added, what errors may be introduced, how the errors can be corrected before decision making, what about cognitive load for healthcare professionals? How to measure the improvement due to context-awareness? How to personalize healthcare applications? Can context and preferences be matched well without any conflicts/side-effects? In this chapter, we address some of these questions and show how context-awareness can help healthcare services.

11.2 Context and Context Awareness

In this section, context and context awareness are discussed along with ways to acquire context information and related challenges.

11.2.1 Context

Context is an important notion in pervasive computing and is also known as circumstances, situation, conditions, surroundings, or environment. The context is any information that can be used to characterize the situation of an entity, which is a person, place, or object that is considered relevant to the interaction between a user and an application, including the user and applications themselves [1]. Context is the set of environmental states and setting that either determines an application's behavior, also known as active context or in which an application event occurs and is interesting to the user, also known as passive context. By including context, the richness of communications can be increased and more useful services can be designed. Context can be explicitly or implicitly indicated by the user, but one of the major goals of context research is to reduce user efforts. The primary context types are location, identity, time, and activity and are used to determine "why". The context can even be further divided among low-level such as time, temperature, and bandwidth and high-level contexts such as complex user activity. Most of these fit under physical context, and then there is something called social context, which may be very rich, but leads to additional complexity [3]. The social context may include user's traits, interests, preferences, if he is alone, who the others are. The context may also include person's emotional/physical states and past actions/history, thus context may depend on both stored (past) information and current information. Context and context-awareness have been addressed by several researchers [1-4, 6-14].

11.2.2 Context Classification

One of the earliest works in context-aware computing involved the classification based on proximate selection of nearby objects, automatic contextual reconfiguration of components, contextual information and commands or different results based on the context, and context-triggered actions such as IF-THEN rules to specify how the adaptation should occur [8]. Another work developed a taxonomy of context-aware features: contextual sensing, contextual adaptation, contextual resource discovery and contextual augmentation, or the ability to associate digital data with a user's context [9]. These have helped in defining various aspects of context-aware computing and necessary actions to perform different activities. More work can be done in creating a classification of the current and emerging context-aware applications and how different set of actions are performed in each application. Some work can also be done in designing new classification system suited for pervasive healthcare.

11.2.3 Context Acquisition

Three types of context acquisitions are possible [7].

1. Sensed context: this type of information is acquired by the mean of physical or software sensors such as temperature, pressure, lighting and noise level.
2. Derived context: this kind of contextual information can be computed on the fly. The most illustrative examples are time and date.
3. Context explicitly provided: For example, user's preferences, when they are explicitly communicated by the user to the requesting application.

In general, there are multiple sources where context information can be acquired:
1. Sensors (ambient, location, health)
2. Information sources (preferences, info on applications and usage, user history, patient's history)
3. Miscellaneous (current network traffic, special conditions in user's surroundings, closest place of interest, distance to a hospital)

It is very important that context-based systems filter any unnecessary information (or too much information) to allow for more effective use of context information or more effective operation of systems as more relevant information can be put together. The filtering may be facilitated if the specific set of information, needed for context acquisition, is known in advance.

There are several challenges in acquiring context in mobile environment. Resource limitations make minimizing context acquisition a practical need, while the uncertainty inherent to the mobile environment makes missing context values a major concern [12]. The authors have used a mechanism based on Bayesian network learning on a restaurant recommender system to show that the mechanism can accurately discover causal dependencies among context, thereby enabling the effective identification of the minimal set of important context for a specific user and task, as well as providing highly accurate recommendations even when context values are missing [12].

One of the challenges is to deal with uncertainty in context. Probabilistic logic, Fuzzy logic, and Bayesian networks can be used in handling uncertainty in different situations. Probabilistic logic involves using probabilities to indicate truth values of statements, as opposed to just 0 or 1 to indicate false or true [21]. This allows it to handle uncertainty, but increases the computational complexity. Bayesian networks are graphical models to represent all variables and their probabilistic independencies [22]. These can handle uncertainty, especially when there are causal relationships between events. Probabilistic logic is useful when the precise knowledge of events' probabilities is known. Fuzzy logic is a multi-valued logic to deal with reasoning that is approximate rather than precise [23]. The degree of truth of a statement can vary between 0 and 1. Fuzzy logic is useful for representing imprecise notions. Both probabilistic and fuzzy logic are useful in scenarios where it is difficult to train a Bayesian network [13]. These three different methods have been incorporated in Gaia, a distributed middleware system. More details on the model for uncertain contexts and how Gaia handles uncertainty and various reasoning mechanisms can be found in [13]. Gaia handles uncertainty in three broad areas: sensing context information, inferring context information, and enabling applications to use uncertain context information. The authors state that highly critical applications require context information with a high level of confidence before they can take action, whereas less critical applications can operate with less certain context information [13]. It should be mentioned that additional complexities and processing requirements of Probabilistic logic, fuzzy logic and Bayesian networks may exceed the limits of many smaller devices and may have to be supported by more powerful devices.

11.2.4 Context Modeling

The contextual information can be modeled in several different ways using data structures that fall into the following categories [2]:

- Key-value pairs: environmental variable as the key and the value of the variable holding the contextual data
- Tagged encoding: context are modeled as tags and corresponding fields
- OO Model: the contextual information is embedded as the states of the object and the object provides methods to access and modify the states. Key value-pairs and tagged encoding can be used to represent context information in the embedded states.
- Logic-based model: context data are expressed as facts in a rule-based system, where new rules can be added as well as submit queries to the database of contextual information.
- Layered model: Raw contextual data is in first layer, the second layer "Cue" gathers these data and outputs a symbolic or sub-symbolic value, while a set of possible values for each cue are defined. Each cue is dependent on single sensor, but multiple cues can be calculated from the data of one sensor. The third layer "context" is derived from the available cues across all sensors.

The context information can be kept centralized, such as by using a centralized context-server to provide contextual information to the applications and also to monitor context changes and send events to interested applications. In distributed implementation, the context information is held at several places and can be implemented using context trigger (condition and action), agents, and multicast for location queries and possible responses [2]. This could also lead to context processing at one or multiple places, if needed.

11.2.5 Context Awareness

The basic ideas behind context awareness are to create "pro-active" and "smart" operation of devices and objects surrounding us by minimizing user efforts and interactions, creating a level of intelligence in the systems, adding adaptability and effective decision making, and increasing the level of customization and personalization for users. Context-awareness is also interpreted as adaptive, responsive, or context-sensitive. In the literature, there are several definitions of context-awareness, ranging from very general to very restrictive. A system is context-aware if it uses context to provide relevant information and/or services to the user, where relevancy depends on the user's task [1]. Thus, context-aware systems have the ability to discover and react to changes in their environment. The keywords are environment, including people, places or objects relevant to the use of application, discover and react. The context includes who (identity), what (activity), where (location), when (temporal) and why (reasoning for behavior and actions). Discovery involves sensing of the entities in the environment. Personalization allows a user to specify his/her preferences, passive context-awareness includes sensing and presentation of changes in context to the user without automatic changes, and active context-awareness involves automatic changes. Some context-aware systems expect the users to provide all information and some not relying on users at all even when making potential mistakes in deriving the context or adapting to changes in context [2]. Figure 11.1 shows the steps in context-awareness, where it is broken into three phases of information, context and adaptation.

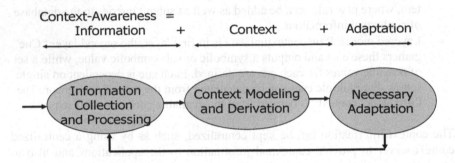

Fig. 11.1 The Steps in Context-awareness

Context awareness can enhance or customize the application behavior to be more personalized for their users. Context information for an application is every thing that could change the behavior of the application like the location, user preferences, environment or properties of connectivity. For context aware applications running on mobile devices, it is vital to deal with the dynamically changing environments and to efficiently exploit the context information within limited resources of the device and mobile communication system. A context dissemination middleware based on a mobile Web Services framework is presented in [11].

In context-aware systems, application autonomy can reduce interactions with users, ease the use of the system, and decrease the user distractions, but it can also take away some control from the user. A better balanced may be achieved by making users aware of reasons for application adaptations by selectively revealing aspects of the application state, such as context information, user preference information and adaptation logic used in decision making processes [10]. Assuming users have some expertise, they may be able to correct undesirable actions by changing context information or preferences appropriately. A survey of what has been done in user control and application autonomy in context-aware systems and requirements for future context-aware systems is presented in [10]. More work is needed on designing, evaluating and comparing techniques for presenting context information to users. This could also include identifying the appropriate individual and combined modes of presentation for different pieces and overall context information. Work is also needed on how to modify (or override) context-aware systems when one or more unexpected actions arise or user requirements change with time. The context-aware systems could be programmed to treat certain unexpected actions as emergency, while ignoring some actions.

To provide monitoring service of arbitrary context information, a rule description (policy) language has been designed. The paper presents an exemplary application in the health care domain to demonstrate the use of the middleware [11]. The proposed middleware provides the base functionalities for mobile devices to publish their context information, and in addition subscribe to the context information published by their mobile peers [11].

11.2.6 Approaches for Context-awareness

With context awareness becoming possible and even desirable in almost every object surrounding us, including sofa, kitchen items, appliances, cars, computers, bed, washer-drawer, there has been some work on identifying approaches for building context-awareness. There are two main approaches [14]. In self-supported context awareness, designers build the ability to perceive context, reason with it, and act accordingly into the device or its dedicated hardware support. In infrastructure-supported context awareness, designers obtain context aware capabilities by harnessing a hardware and software infrastructure external to and associated with the device's space. Such an infrastructure might implement the context-aware behavior of specific objects and devices or act as a general context-aware infrastructure [14]. In self-supported context-awareness, objects are usually equipped with sensors to achieve information. This also reduces dependency on external infrastructure, however, implementing this requires embedding sensors unobtrusively, reasoning with the context efficiently and accurately, and enabling appropriate actions. In infrastructure-supported context awareness, the infrastructure first receives the contextual information and, if appropriate, reasons with it. It then either issues commands or feeds contextual information to the application or artifact for appropriate actions. Finally, the application might provide feedback to the infrastructure. And, just as the same infrastructure can support many context-aware artifacts, the same artifact might be supported by different infrastructures at different times (for example, when the artifact changes location) [14]. An infrastructure can help link inputs from new sensors to new kinds of responsive artifacts, enabling some very interesting context-aware behaviors such as a wall painted with smart paint might change color to our emotions and movements [14].

Another example could be reminder for medications or notification for one of several conditions.

11.2.7 Challenges in Context-awareness

There are several challenges in context-awareness paradigm. First, it is not yet widely adopted, possibly due to a lack of reusable architectures/mechanisms for context acquisition and storage. Also, most existing systems do not allow easy inclusion of new contexts. Such work will involve substantial modification of the systems along with added complexity. Scalability and privacy of context-aware applications are some more unaddressed challenges [7].

11.3 Context in Healthcare

The healthcare area, especially pervasive healthcare, is highly suitable for using context-aware systems in delivery of healthcare services. Here are some reasons why context-awareness is more useful in healthcare. First, there are a large number of situations and related tasks; potential for cognitive overload; mobility of patients, healthcare professionals and some equipments; limited financial and human resources; and the need to cut cost while improving the quality of service to an increased number of people. Although context-awareness infrastructure including more complex devices and software will add to the total cost, the reduced number of medical errors and the ability to more effectively utilize healthcare resources should lead to reduced cost. Then, the expectation to access, process, and modify healthcare information anywhere using handheld devices is another reason to use context-awareness. The need to support the human-computer interaction is also important in pervasive healthcare. In some sense, pervasive healthcare may be the "killer" application for context-awareness.

Healthcare professionals can provide some environmental and initializing information for context-awareness in comprehensive health monitoring systems. But, in practice, it may be a challenge to collect information from users, process and filter, and put together only relevant information, which may be subject to change.

11.3.1 Summary of Work in Healthcare

The use of context and context-awareness in healthcare is an emerging area and there has been only limited work so far. We summarize some of the representative work here. A wearable healthcare system, called LifeMinder, derives context information using patient's photos, voice, posture and actions [15]. The wearable prototype can sense pulse waves and user actions/postures and captures contextual photos and voice, which are then stored on a website for subsequent retrieval. An acceleration sensor detects the user's vertical and forward horizontal acceleration. A microcontroller uses a context sensing method and acceleration data to calculate user's action and postures (walking, running, standing, sitting, and lying). A camera and microphone record still pictures and ambient sounds. LifeMinder detects high-pressure stressful states from high-pulse rate over 90bpm with the user's context information [15]. It collects such data and also computes high-pressure ratio as the sum of time of the high-pressure state/total time and can be used to relate to the conditions of a person such as little nervous, relax, in-presentation, and desk-work [15].

The application of context-aware computing has been suggested in [4]. The vision and design guidelines along with summary from meetings with healthcare workers focus on context-aware pill container and context-aware hospital bed, designed to react and adapt to their context. The context-aware bed has RFID sensors to identify the patient, staff and physicians and a display to show any relevant information and warning for some incorrect actions [4]. The patient can use the bedside computer for Internet access. The location and identity of the pill container are supported using RFID. The context-aware pill container reacts and adapts to the changes in its environment and by using an authentication system (such as finger prints), it supports proper dose administration [4]. The context-awareness is useful for user-interface navigation. The use of context-awareness for immediate action may be annoying when the sensed context is incorrect, but a user could be given several choices (suggested course of action) and the user could accept one or more or could reject all [4].

Context-aware MobileWard is designed to support nurses in conducting morning procedures in a hospital ward [3]. It discovers and reacts autonomously according to changes in the environment and provides information and services to the user based on the user's task. It integrates both temporal, such as time schedules, and spatial, such as different wards, information. The design of prototype is based on ethnographic studies identifying mobility and collaboration. It holds promise but may add potential interaction problems when users are mobile and working in a professional environment. Many times as the context changed, the system reacted and moved away from the information that a user was still reading [3]. Additional work can be done in decision making on when to react to changes. This could include postponing the action if the user is still reading. The system could ask the user to provide an input or sense the context of the user, or trying to find what does the user want. It could be personalized in setting up the "reactions" of the system when the context changes.

Healthcare professionals are involved in a variety of tasks and processes and their informational needs vary based on their location, time and the involved activity. The knowledge of their current activity may assist in deciding which of the healthcare professionals should be reached for some medical tasks or decision

making. Some work has been done in context based estimation of activity performed by a healthcare professional [25]. Using a neural network, trained with
hours of data, the authors show that about 75% accuracy can be obtained in estimating the current activity a person is involved in [25].

Many people, normally older adults or those in geriatric years, may suffer from
dementia. One of the symptoms is the agitated behavior, including body movements and certain speech patterns. With an increasing number of such patients in
US and other countries due to the population aging, there will be a need for detailed and continuous monitoring for dementia. One way to derive objective outcomes is to use certain behavior patterns [16]. The work involves a context aware
patient data collection system (CAPDCS), which utilizes the features extracted
from each sensor modality. Using a scale based on body movements and speech
patterns including repetitive, negative and loud words, the tool attempt to identify
the degree of agitation experienced by a demented person. The authors reported
high (90%) accuracy for simple actions and low (50-60%) accuracy for complex
behavior [16].

Hospitals are highly desirable places for deploying ubiquitous computing as their
workers experience a high level of mobility and different types of workers may
need to look for different pieces of information. Hospital information systems
(HISs) that provide access to electronic patient records could provide accurate and
timely information to hospital staff in medical decision-making. One way to do
this is by utilizing public displays in conjunction with mobile devices in displaying the needed information. Public displays become aware of the presence of physicians and nurses in their vicinity and adapt to provide users with personalized,
relevant information. An agent-based architecture allows the integration of proactive components that offer information relevant to the case at hand, either from
medical guidelines or previous similar cases [17]. Authors explore the use of interactive public displays in hospitals and their integration into a context-aware
mobile computing infrastructure developed for hospitals. The authors noted that
the medical staff need to locate relevant documents, such as patient' records, laboratory results, and forms to be filled, locate patients and colleagues, and locate and
track the availability of devices, such as medical equipment and beds, which are
moved within the hospital. With adequate support to estimate the context of work,
context-aware systems can deliver information that is relevant to the user's location, identity, and/or role [17].

The context can also be used in managing access to patient's information, such as
those stored in electronic patient record (EPR). The design of proper models for
authorization and access control for EPR is essential to wide scale use of EPR in
large health organizations. The authors propose a contextual role-based access
control authorization model aiming to increase the patient privacy and the confidentiality of patient data, whereas being flexible enough to consider specific cases
[18]. Contextual authorizations use the environmental information available at access time, like user/patient relationship, in order to decide whether a user is allowed to access an EPR resource. One of the major challenges is to devise au-

thorization and access control models capable of supporting exceptional cases (such as emergencies), taking into account any contextual or conditional information [18].

In the healthcare field, biomechanical data generated by advanced technical devices are not well utilized. To improve this, a method has been proposed to support clinicians, especially those in orthopedics, in the contextual interpretation of biomechanical data [19]. The authors characterize temporal biomechanical data by means of fuzzy space–time windows and to induce fuzzy decision trees to map the biomechanical and clinical data related to patients. The authors also present a method for objectively explaining a given clinical characteristic of a particular patient; this method is derived using the fuzzy rule base generated from the trees and a satisfiability measure [19]. By supporting clinicians during the biomechanical data interpretation process, the method helps them take the objective biomechanical measurements in the medical practice into account, particularly in orthopedics. It can also make subjective evaluations more objective by mapping subjective and objective data [19].

Detection of falls, especially in elderly, is an important healthcare requirement. In the current scenarios, it may be hours or even days before such someone finds out and come for help, especially for people who are living by themselves. It has been known that several major health complications could arise due to falls and the delayed response could increase the severity of such conditions. There has been some work in automatic detection of falls based on detection/estimation of posture and pressure on sensor-equipped floors. However, the accuracy of such detection varies and may not detect all falls. The use of visual fall detection along with context information has been proposed in [24]. The context model is extensive as it integrates different types of knowledge in assessing falls including patient's general condition, orientation and location, and the time and duration of patient's inactivity [24].

11.3.2 Challenges in Pervasive Healthcare

Some major challenges in using context-awareness in pervasive healthcare are (a) derivation of context, which could be evolving at different rates in different healthcare services, (b) the need to adapt to changes in context as it evolves and (c) corrective actions when something goes wrong in a context-aware system involved in healthcare delivery. Additionally, there are some limitations of context and context-awareness in pervasive healthcare. In some healthcare services, the description of a situation by using what (activity), who (identity), where (location) and when (time) may not enough, where more richness and higher reliability are required. This could include how (process), with whom (source), and so what (needed action). This will either increase the complexity of context-aware system or will result in higher chance of error in the delivery of healthcare services. The increased complexity could also lead to a slower operation of systems, not desirable for some services, such as emergency services in pervasive healthcare.

11.4. Context in Health Monitoring

In healthcare environment, in addition to location, identity, time and activity, the context types may also include current medications, handicaps, and current environment and may relate with a person's identity and/or location, but likely to change with time. In wireless health monitoring, healthcare professionals will make decisions based on knowledge derived from multiple set of informational items such as patient's medical history, current vital signs, medical knowledge, and specific patient conditions.

Comprehensive health monitoring requires that monitoring be autonomous, reliable and error free. The autonomous operation will allow monitoring in situations where a patient is not able to intervene in the monitoring process. In addition, the monitoring should be personalized and scalable. Personalization will improve the overall medical decision making, while scalability of monitoring systems will allow the monitoring of more patients or more frequent monitoring of the same number of patients. These issues have not been addressed in health monitoring research and certainly more work is needed before comprehensive wireless health monitoring becomes a reality. These requirements can be supported by employing context awareness in the monitoring systems. Context awareness will allow the monitoring systems to adapt to a patient's current needs without his/her intervention, create monitoring messages with suitable priority level, and adapt to network traffic. The use of context along with a range of information on a patient will improve the correctness of medical decision making. The adaptation could also include balancing a patient's requirements and network traffic. The use of context could lead to multi-point enhancements, including monitoring devices, networks, and healthcare professional devices, to improve the end-to-end reliability. The use of traffic management techniques, employing context-based priority and use of live and stored health information, could improve infrastructure scalability.

Thus, comprehensive wireless health monitoring system should be actively context-aware, which will also aid in a better decision making by healthcare professionals on patient's current conditions and healthcare needs. In health monitoring, users can be patients whose primary task is being monitored for one or more health conditions and receive necessary medical attention, or healthcare professionals, whose primary task is to receive current and accurate information on monitored patients and perform decision making on patients' conditions and required care.

One of the major applications of context-awareness in healthcare would be to create a "virtual" follow up appointment with a healthcare professional. This will involve collecting and transmitting accurate and useful information to healthcare professional as if the patient was in an actual follow up appointment. For example, if a patient has been in treatment for depression, the physician would normally ask the patient on a follow up visit if they have been taking medicine regularly, sleeping well, physically active and exercising. Such information can be programmed in health monitoring system to look for symptoms and contextual-clues as a healthcare professional may do in person follow up appointment.

11.4.1 Context from the Type of Monitoring

In very simple terms, context may indicate the type of monitoring. Comprehensive health monitoring could cover scenarios involving patients with different levels of mobility, locations, timeliness of monitoring, and, reactive vs proactive monitoring (Figure 11.2). In passive monitoring, the vital signs are recorded for a subsequent analysis by healthcare professionals, while active monitoring involves generation, transmission and analysis of live vital signs and related information. As it can be observed that the resource requirements for these two types of monitoring will differ significantly. The monitoring types can be further divided in continuous or event-driven, based on whether the health monitoring is continuous or event-driven such as passage of time or patient intervention. This context of time will lead to support different monitoring applications and scenarios, and will require different level of processing, storage, and network resources. The health monitoring can also focus on stationary or mobile patients, essentially addressing the context of mobility. For health monitoring, a patient could wear a wearable computing system such as Smart Shirt or its LifeShirt version, use a hand-held device with sensors, or be a part of some smart environment. The most demanding is the active continuous monitoring involving mobile patients wearing monitoring devices and needing pervasive coverage without their intervention or inputs. This type of monitoring should be carefully chosen or the health monitoring systems could spend considerable time and resources on providing this most demanding service to cases that could have been supported by another simpler monitoring type.

These variations of health monitoring types require different quality of service. The quality of service here implies the level of service quality that should be provided by the underlying hardware and software infrastructure for health monitoring. The infrastructure includes monitoring devices and software, networks and devices and software used by healthcare professionals. In some sense, the context information for the type of monitoring can be mapped into quality of service (QoS) requirement. To facilitate this mapping, several QoS attributes for healthcare, or more specifically monitoring services, are needed. To address this, we define several attributes, termed together as Healthcare Quality of Service (H-QoS), shown in Table 11.1.

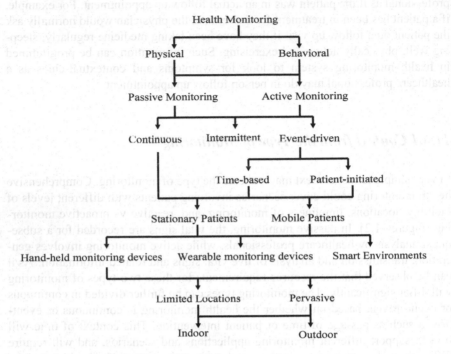

Fig. 11.2 Context from the Type of Monitoring

Table 11.1 Healthcare quality of service

Type of H-QoS	Attributes	Importance	The role of context
Patient-centric (P-QoS)	Reliability of message delivery	When patient's sign are out of normal range (emergency cases)	Context information can be used to prioritize messages to improve this QoS
	Monitoring delays		
Network-centric (N-QoS)	Message throughput (number of message transmitted)	When network capacity is limited (as in wireless networks) or when the monitoring traffic is routine	Context information on the type of monitoring and patients could be used in optimizing this QoS
	Scalability in terms of number of patients supported		
Healthcare professional-centric (HP-QoS)	The number of correct medical decisions	When complex and life-saving decisions have to made (emergency cases)	Could improve the correctness of medical decisions
	The cognitive load of healthcare professionals		Focusing on most important information could reduce the cognitive load

11.4.2 Context from Patient Records and Stored Information

In simple terms, some of the patient information may be available as part of EMR (Electronic Medical Record), which includes at least the following four pieces of information for a complete implementation: (a) computerized orders for prescriptions, (b) computerized orders for tests, (c) reporting of test results, and (d) physician notes. Currently, it is estimated that 25% of the physicians in US use it, but only about 10% use it fully. Several countries have proposed deadlines for a version of EMR, EHR (Electronic Health Record) or EPR (Electronic Patient Record). These include Year-2010 for UK and EHR 2014 as the US deadline. The current obstacles are cost, disruption to care, interoperability between different systems, privacy and legal aspects, older medical records, and technology challenges.

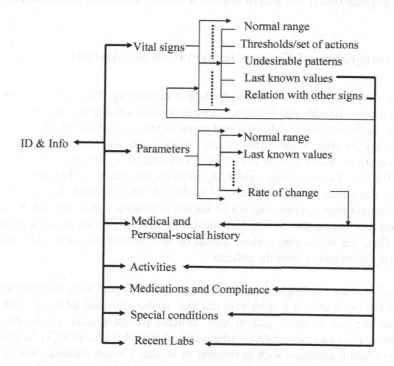

Fig. 11.3 Representation of Patient's Information

The use of EMR/EHR/EPR is driven by the need to reduce medical errors, which could result in wrong diagnosis and drug interaction problems. These occur due to a lack of correct and complete information at the location and time it is needed. There is a need to make the necessary patient/health information available at "any place anytime". In general, overall quality and healthcare coverage can be enhanced by reducing inefficiencies and improve handling of medical information. However, problems in the electronic records or lack of access to the records, especially in emergencies could lead to much worse situations.

Figure 11.3 shows how medical information can be represented for individual patients to achieve a significantly high degree of personalization. Although some of the information can be obtained from EMR/EHR/EPR, the representation here is richer and information can easily be utilized in deriving and using context information. The vital signs are defined with multiple thresholds, set of actions, undesirable patterns, and inter-relationship between multiple vital signs. The representation of medical information will be helpful for designing a comprehensive health monitoring system by utilizing both stored and live information. This along with the patient's current context (surroundings, patient's current activity, and emotional/physical states) will lead to suitable actions by healthcare professionals.

11.5 Integration of Context Information and Details

Use of the context would be useful for health monitoring. This will allow the offering of most suitable and useful services to patients without wasting network resources as the number of false positive cases, where system incorrectly detects an emergency situation without having one, may be reduced without increasing the false negatives, where system fails to detect an emergency situation when there is one. The use of context may potentially improve the quality of life with reduced anxiety and ability to get most suitable healthcare when needed. The use of context in monitoring services may not be known to patients and it may not matter as patients may not be able to help the monitoring system with all possible information. Thus, the monitoring system should be able operate autonomously without requiring intervention from the patients.

Example 1: One vital sign is represented as an ECG signal with multiple waves, which follows a certain pattern with duration (pulse rate) and intensity. Any significant changes in wave pattern may indicate patient-specific cardio-vascular problems. For example, relative variations in different waves in ECG indicates a range of health problems such as missing or weaker P wave indicates atrial problems affecting blood flow to the heart. A large increase in Q wave with respect to overall QRS indicates myocardial infraction (heart attack), while inverted T wave indicates ischemia. In addition to the current values of vital signs and patient-specific thresholds, the health monitoring system, to differentiate a multitude of situations, could also utilize physical location, physiological and emotional states, personal health history, and, current activities. In addition, in case of the availability of sensors, such information could also be utilized with patient's history of medical information. The current ECG values along with context information will improve the medical decision making of healthcare professionals.

Example 2: After the vital signs are acquired, threshold and pattern-based processing is done to determine the level of emergency and a suitable action is taken, such as generation of a transmission event with a certain priority. A set of rules will be specified for a device, specific to a patient and his/her history and current condition, by a healthcare professional for comprehensive monitoring. These rules will lead to a more accurate generation of "alerts" as more detailed information, context of the patient and his/her surroundings, and medical history will be included. A patient suffering from Chronic Obstructive Pulmonary Disease (COPD) where breathing is difficult due to lung damage would need to have vital signs of ECG and respiration rate closely monitored. For this patient, an "alert" can be generated by using COPD context and the two mentioned vital signs (when out-of-range). The rules can be modified as necessary by healthcare professionals, patient's attendant, or intelligent devices with significant processing abilities. To manage complexity, the number of possible contexts can be kept to a certain value for a patient, or most likely context can be considered. For implementation, devices without complex processing functionality could either include simple decision making and generate "alerts" or in the simplest case allow healthcare professionals to analyze all of the vital signs themselves without any processing help from devices. These emergency messages must be reliably delivered to healthcare professionals with minimal delays and without any message corruption.

Example 3: The use of air quality can also be used in deriving the context, especially for people suffering from asthma and other pulmonary illnesses, and one or more cardiac conditions. The air quality could be obtained from sensors and/or weather reports (Figure 11.4). This along with age of the patients, especially very young and very old, current location with outdoor-much worse and indoor-less worse, and any history of pulmonary problems could be integrated and transmitted to healthcare professionals for medical decision making. In some cases, the derived context could be used to send a proactive reminder to older people, with pulmonary and cardiac problems, living at home or in an assisted living.

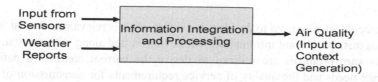

Fig. 11.4 Using Information from Multiple Sources for Context Input

In general, context or a set of filtered and relevant information such as <location, activity, time, identity and social context-like living alone, medical history, environmental variables, and labs>, which is presented along with current vital signs and parameters to healthcare professionals for medical decision making (option 1). In more advanced scenarios with sophisticated monitoring devices, it may be possible to integrate context with vital signs and parameters to generate possible medical problems and then sent to healthcare professionals for final medical decision (option 2). In some cases, option 1 could be used, but if requested by healthcare professionals, option 2 may be offered. Certainly, option 2 requires more intelligence, processing, and storage from health monitoring systems than option 1.

11.5.1 Collection of Information

The type of information that could be collected include the type of health monitoring, vital signs, prescribed medicines, sensory information, activities, environmental variables, and patient history. The information on missing doses, recent labs, known handicaps, and unusual conditions will also be very useful in health monitoring. The information may come from multiple sources such as sensors, wearable and portable computers, some databases that may have information on the patient or from patient's input in some cases.

There are many challenges before such systems can be implemented. These include how often the information needs to be collected, when is some information too old or not useful, what should be the granularity level, and how much traffic will be created to and from the monitoring system? Also, what if some information is old, not reliable, missing, or just plain wrong? How would the monitoring system deal with it? What is the Minimum Set of Information (MSI) required for reliable monitoring results? Is it same for normal, abnormal, or emergency cases? In practice, even a single (or limited) piece of highly unusual information must result in generation of an "alert".

11.5.2 Filtering and Processing of Information

The protocols are also used to decide what information is relevant and what is not. Based on this, all relevant information will be transmitted along with context. The context-aware protocols are utilized to derive the current context of patient's healthcare needs and the quality of service requirements for transmission of vital signs (Figure 11.5). More specifically, context can be utilized to derive the QoS requirements by differentiating among the multiple possibilities represented by absolute values of vital signs and thresholds. Thus context-awareness can lead to better derivation of the level of emergency for a monitored patient. It is important how the context information is presented for decision making to a healthcare professional. The context-generation protocols are designed to *assist* and not *replace* the medical decision making by healthcare professionals. Therefore, if the context is incorrect or there is problem, the monitoring system would allow the healthcare professional to request more information and make a better decision. The protocols can be stored and processed in the health monitoring devices that a patient can carry or wear as a part of smart clothing. The context-generation protocols can be modified to work with incomplete and/or missing information in deriving the patient's context and healthcare needs. The context generated will then be transmitted over networks along with live patient information. In some cases, based on the current status and the level and type of disability, a patient could correct the "derived" context, which will improve the accuracy of health monitoring; however, this is not a requirement as the system is designed to operate in an autonomous environment.

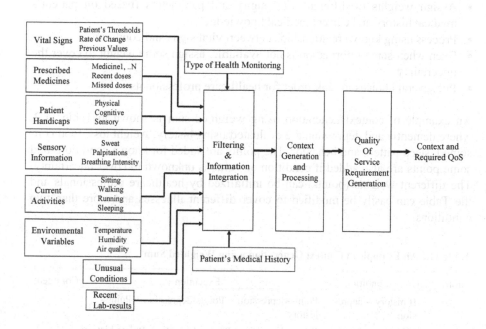

Fig. 11.5 Patient's Healthcare Context and QoS Requirement

11.5.3 Context Generation using Weighted Sum

The context can be generated using weighted sum of different input variables to generate probabilities, which are then mapped into one or more likely contexts. For such context generation, the monitoring system needs to know different weights, needs to process all the available information, and needs to account for information which is not available or reliable such as old lab reports. This type of context generation could result in one or more possible contexts, could lead to some errors due to processing, and current weights, and may require more complex devices. Weighted-sum context can lead to very personalized WPM due to the use of personalized weights, thresholds, and possibility of learning from previous outcomes and errors to improve future accuracy, and can help a healthcare professional in medical decision making.

The steps could include

- Assign weights to different vital signs and parameters (based on patient's medical history and current medical knowledge)
- Process using known relationships between vital signs and conditions
- Even when some information is not available, assign some weight to cover the uncertainty
- Put several choices in rank-order for healthcare professionals

An example of context generation using weighted sum is shown in Table 11.2, where dementia and depression are evaluated using history, weight loss, food consumed, sleep pattern and behavior. The points are added for known conditions and some points are also added if condition or value is unknown to cover uncertainty. The different weights (points) can be initialized by healthcare professionals and the Table can easily be modified to cover different illnesses and more than two conditions.

Table 11.2 An Example of Context Generation using Weighted Sum

Information	Condition	Execution	Comment
	If history = depression	Points-depression = Points-depression + Points-history	
History	If history = dementia	Points-dementia = Points-dementia + Points-history	
	If history = unknown	Points-depression = Points-depression + Points-history-unknown	Add some weight to cover uncertainty
		Points-dementia = Points-dementia + Points-history-unknown	
Weight loss	If (2weekweightloss>weight-threshold)	Points-depression = Points-depression + Points-weightloss	
		Points-dementia = Points-dementia + Points-	

		weightloss	
	If (2weekweightloss= unknown)	Points-depression = Points-depression + Points-weightloss-unknown	Add some weight to cover un-certainty
		Points-dementia = Points-dementia + Points-weightloss-unknown	
Food Consumed	If (foodcon-sumed<food-threshold)	Points-depression = Points-depression + Points-food	
		Points-dementia = Points-dementia + Points-food	
	If (foodconsumed= unknown)	Points-depression = Points-depression + Points-food-unknown	Add some weight to cover un-certainty
		Points-dementia = Points-dementia + Points-food-unknown	
Sleep Pat-tern	If (sleeppat-tern<acceptable-level)	Points-depression = Points-depression + Points-sleep	
		Points-dementia = Points-dementia + Points-sleep	
	If (sleeppattern= un-known)	Points-depression = Points-depression + Points-sleep-unknown	Add some weight to cover un-certainty
		Points-dementia = Points-dementia + Points-sleep-unknown	
Behavior	If (behavior= violent)	Points-depression = Points-depression + Points-violent	
		Points-dementia = Points-dementia + Points-violent	
	If (behavior= un-known)	Points-depression = Points-depression + Points-violent-unknown	Add some weight to cover un-certainty
		Points-dementia = Points-dementia + Points-violent-unknown	
Overall Output		Context (history, weightloss, foodconsumed, sleep-pattern, behavior)	To pro-duce final output
		Rank order (depression, dementia)	

Another example of context generation using weighted sum is presented here. The information on patient's activities, medical history, and vital signs variations are included with their relative weights, personalized to the patient, to create context-aware wireless health monitoring. For implementation, the relative weights are expressed as points, and emergency level is derived based on the sum of all points (Figure 11.6). For example, vital signs are compared with different "personalized" thresholds and points are added. The rate of change of a vital sign is compared against a threshold rate and if the vital sign exceeds it, some points are added. If the current activity is resting, then some more points are added to reflect that any abnormality in vital signs is not due to the current activity such as exercise. Many more factors can be added to improve the accuracy of emergency detection and the weights (points) can be modified to reflect changes in patient conditions and the need to adjust the numbers of false positives and false negatives.

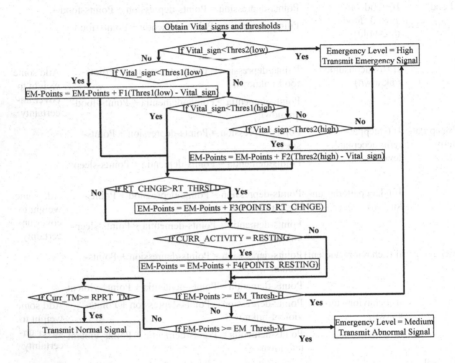

Fig. 11.6 The Protocol Used by Wireless Health Monitoring Device

11.5.4 Context Generation using Set of Rules

Here, sets of conditional statements are used for checking certain combinations for a certain context. For this, monitoring system needs to know the set of rules, needs to check specific conditions, but does not need to process all the available information. This will result in simple Yes or No answer as an outcome of checking one or more possible contexts, but may have problems with missing or unavailable or unreliable information as sometimes some of the conditional statements may fail. It is still possible to make it personalized using patient-specific thresholds, but it can be quicker to just check for one or more problems. Context generation, using set of rules, allows to limit the number of possibilities to manage complexity, processing, and storage for mobile devices. The focus is on the most likely contexts (assist and not replace). An example is shown in Table 11.3 where set of rules are checked against the available information to generate context.

Table 11.3 An Example of Context Generation Using Set of Rules

Condition	Execution	Comment
	Check Activities & Vital Signs	As part of continuous of periodic monitoring
If activity=exercising posture= not fallen down vital signs = higher normal history= no heart problems	Level of emergency = low	The other factors included in the context generation compensate for high normal vital signs.
If activity=sleeping vital signs = higher normal history= known heart problems	Level of emergency = high	The other factors included in the context generation worsen high normal vital signs.

Another example could include mental health monitoring where one of the two sets of conditions could lead to generation of high level of emergency. This is shown in Table 11.4.

Table 11.4 Another Example with Two Sets of Conditions Used

Condition	Execution	Comment
If (behavior= violent)	level of emergency = high	Violent behavior alone is sufficient
If past-history = mental-illness sleep <= sleep-threshold eating <=eating-threshold	level of emergency = high	All the three statements have to be true

So, weighted sum is the preferred method of context-generation in scenarios with missing or incomplete information and set of rules is best for scenarios with most information available. In practice, it can be shown that these two methods of context generation are equivalent. Also, other methods that can account for uncertainty could be included to improve the accuracy of context generation.

11.5.5 Related Issues in Context-management

There are many challenges in context-management. These include how to deal with uncertainty in users' locations, potential inaccuracy in the current location, system's inability to track a patient due to falls, uncovered areas, or one or more failures in the system. These open issues should be addressed in future work. Also, there may be some privacy challenges with context-information unless the monitoring system deletes the context once the service is completed. There are also issues in who can access what patient was doing before needing the help, and how many humans may know or monitor what a patient is doing or was doing at some time.

11.6 From Context-awareness to Health-Awareness

In many cases, the description of a health situation by using multiple constructs of what (activity), who (identity), where (location) and when (time) may be enough for most healthcare services. However, in cases where a higher level of richness and reliability is required, additional constructs such as how (process), from whom (source), and so what (needed action) or which could be employed. The use of additional constructs will help identify not only the needs of a patient but will also identify new diseases, sources of bio-terrorism, and the future healthcare needs of many more people. We term the richer level of awareness as "Complete-Awareness". Complete awareness is a new paradigm that adds more richness and complexity in the study of various phenomena and how to improve systems (Figure 11.7). It is suited for healthcare and can also be called health awareness.

There are several challenges in using complete awareness in healthcare or health monitoring services. These include questions like when to use it? How much more benefits can be expected by healthcare systems that support complete-awareness? How much complexity does it add to the underlying infrastructure for pervasive healthcare? What happens when not all information is available? Then, more estimation may have to be done to reduce uncertainty while increasing the correctness of the derived values. Can complete-aware systems handle "incomplete" information or information which may not be reliably current? How to update it when some information components change? Certainly, much more work is required before complete awareness becomes an implemented reality; however this does have the potential to move healthcare services to an unprecedented level of intelligence and quality.

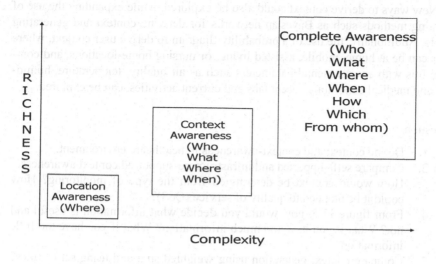

Fig. 11.7 Moving from Context-awareness to Complete Awareness

11.7 Summary and Future

For fulfilling the vision of context-awareness in wireless health monitoring, more work is needed in designing and implementing context-aware protocols and conducting performance evaluation of health monitoring system. Having only a finite number of allowable contexts can ensure reduced complexity in context-awareness. The future research must also address systems that are not only passively context-aware, but can actively adapt to context changes by modifying services to patients and healthcare professionals. This could lead to scenarios where trade-off between the quality of wireless health monitoring and the level of complexity due to context-awareness must have to be considered. More work can also be done in personalization and assignment of weights to different conditions in deriving context. With increasing medical knowledge, further generation of conditional statements or set of rules for context will be required. The reduction in medical errors is one of the fundamental goals of health monitoring and use of context is primarily driven by the need to reduce a range of errors that may be caused by difficulties in medical decision making by healthcare professionals. The focus of context could be to minimize the number of false positives in health monitoring and reduction in unnecessary care. Even more importantly, the goal of zero false negatives and ideally no cases of missing the needed healthcare must be attempted.

New ways to derive context could also be explored, while expanding the use of existing methods such as Bayesian networks for deriving context and generating alerts. Additionally, the use of a probability diagram to derive user context, where user can be at home, mobile, assisted living, or nursing home-locations, and combine this with environmental parameters such as air quality, temperature, humidity, and medical conditions, recent labs and current activities, can be explored.

Questions:

1. Define context and context-awareness in healthcare environment.
2. Compare self-supported and infrastructure-supported context awareness.
3. How would context be determined from the type of monitoring? How could it be mapped to quality of service (QoS)?
4. From figure 11.5, how would you decide what information is useful and not? What if you have too much information? What if you have too little information
5. Compare context generation using weighted sum and using set of rules? Can you show that these two are equivalent in some cases?
6. How would complete awareness or health awareness be used in detecting an epidemic or spread of disease?

References

[1] Dey A, Abowd G (1999) Towards a better understanding of context and context-awareness. Tech Report, GIT-GVU-99-22, Georgia Institute of Technology, June

[2] Chen G, Kotz D (2000) A survey of context-aware mobile computing research. Tech Report, TR2000-381, Dartmouth Computer Science Department

[3] Skov M, Hoegh R (2006) Supporting information access in a hospital ward by a context-aware mobile electronic patient record. Journal of Perv. and Ubiq. Computing, 10: 205-214

[4] Bardram J (2004) Applications of context-aware computing in hospital work-examples and design principles. In Proc. ACM Symposium on Applied Computing

[5] Stefanov D, Bien Z, Bang W (2004) The smart house for older persons and persons with physical disabilities: structure, technology, arrangements, and perspectives. IEEE Transactions on Neural Systems and Rehabilitation Engineering, 12(2): 228-250, June

[6] Helal S, Mann W, Zabadani H, King J, Kaddoura Y, Jensen E (2005) The gator tech smart house: a programmable pervasive space. IEEE Computer, 38(3): 64-74, March

[7] Mostifaoui G, Pasquier-Rocha J, Brkzillon P (2004) Context-aware computing: a guide for the pervasive computing community. IEEE/ACS International Conference on Pervasive Services (ICPS), 39-48

[8] Schilit B, Adams N, Want R (1994) Context-aware computing applications. In Proc. IEEE Workshop on Mobile Computing Systems and Applications, 85-90, December

[9] Pascoe J (1998) Adding generic contextual capabilities to wearable computers. In Proc. Second IEEE International Symposium on Wearable Computers, October

[10] Hardian B, Indulska J, Henricksen K (2006) Balancing autonomy and user control in context-aware systems - a survey. In Proc. Fourth Annual IEEE International Conference on Pervasive Computing and Communications Workshops (PERCOMW'06)

[11] Gehlen G, Aijaz F, Sajjad M, Walke B (2007) A mobile context dissemination middleware. In Proc. IEEE International Conference on Information Technology (ITNG'07)

[12] Yap G, Tan A, Pang H (2006) Discovering causal dependencies in mobile context-aware recommenders. In Proc. IEEE Mobile Data Management Conference

[13] Ranganathan A, Al-Muhtadi J, Campbell R (2004) Reasoning about uncertain contexts in pervasive computing environments. IEEE Pervasive Computing, 3(2): 62-70, April-June

[14] Loke S (2006) Context-aware artifacts: two development approaches. IEEE Pervasive Computing, 5 (2): 48-53, April-June

[15] Suzuki T, Doi M (2001) LifeMinder: an evidence-based wearable healthcare assistant. In Proc. ACM Conference on Human Factors in Computing Systems (CHI)

[16] Biswas J, et.al. (2006) Data collection and feature extraction for a smart ward application. In Proc. IEEE Conference on Emerging Technologies and Factory Automation, 110-115

[17] Favela J, Rodríguez M, Preciado A, González V (2004) Integrating context-aware public displays into a mobile hospital information system. IEEE Transactions on Information Technology in BioMedicine, 8(3): 279-286 September

[18] Motta G, Furuie S (2003) A contextual role-based access control authorization model for electronic patient record. IEEE Transactions on Information Technology in BioMedicine, 7(3): 202-207, September

[19] Roux E, Godillon-Maquinghen A, Caulier P, Bouilland S, Bouttens D (2006) A support method for the contextual interpretation of biomechanical data. IEEE Transactions on Information Technology in BioMedicine, 10(1): 109-118, January

[20] Varshney U (2007) Pervasive healthcare and wireless patient monitoring. ACM/Springer Journal on Mobile Networks and Applications (MONET), 12(2-3):113-127, March

[21] Nilsson, N. J. (1986) Probabilistic logic. Artificial Intelligence 28(1): 71-87

[22] Wikipedia on Bayesian Networks: http://en.wikipedia.org/wiki/Bayesian_network

[23] Wikipedia on Fuzzy Logic: http://en.wikipedia.org/wiki/Fuzzy_logic

[24] Jansen B, Deklerck R (2006) Context aware inactivity recognition for visual fall detection. Proceedings of First International Conference on Pervasive Computing Technologies for Healthcare (IEEE)

[25] Favela J, Tentori M, Castrol L, Gonzalez V, Moran E, Martínez-García A (2006) Estimating hospital work activities in context-aware healthcare applications. Proceedings of First International Conference on Pervasive Computing Technologies for Healthcare (IEEE), Nov.

Chapter 12 Monitoring of Mental Health, Medication and Disability

Abstract Mental health is fast becoming a major challenge worldwide as the incidence of mental illness has been increasing. It is affecting the quality of life as well as job productivity for a large number of people. Just like physical illnesses, people with mental illnesses can be treated and monitored for a range of conditions and provided medical care as and when necessary. In this chapter, we introduce a new field of wireless psychiatry, or a way to address many problems using wireless technologies. This includes comprehensive monitoring of patients for symptoms, behavior, and medication compliance. The monitoring for behavior includes suicidal and homicidal behavior; monitoring for related physical conditions such as sleep patterns and weight loss as part of depression and suicidal behavior; and any weight gain due to inactivity and certain medications. Several examples of mental health monitoring, medication compliance monitoring and disability monitoring are also presented.

12. 1 Introduction

Mental health is a state of successful performance of mental function, resulting in productive activities, fulfilling relationships with other people, and the ability to adapt to change and to cope with adversity [1]. Mental illnesses include all of the known and diagnosable disorders. While some mental illnesses cause relatively mild distress, others result in severe impairment and may require hospitalization [2]. Some major classes of mental illnesses and their examples are shown in Table 12.1. The most common are major depression, bipolar disorder or manic-depressive disorder, Schizophrenia, obsessive-compulsive disorder, panic disorder, substance abuse disorder, post-traumatic stress disorder and dementias such as Alzheimer. A general group of mental illnesses is also known as personality disorders, which is characterized by persistent, inflexible and dysfunctional patterns of thought, action, emotion, and attitude that cause distress in social, job, personal, and family environments [2]. The most common of these types are borderline, histrionic, narcissistic, obsessive-compulsive, and paranoid disorders and may occur with other disorders such as anxiety and depression.

The prevalence of mental illness is about 25% in western countries and is considerably lower in many developing countries. The lower incidence in developing countries could be attributed to better family support, more physically active life, and slower pace of life. However, with ongoing changes in life style, increased

U. Varshney, *Pervasive Healthcare Computing: EMR/EHR, Wireless and Health Monitoring*,
DOI: 10.1007/978-1-4419-0215-3_12,
© Springer Science + Business Media, LLC 2009

259

level of stress, breaking of family structure, and poor diets in developing countries, such difference in the incidence of mental illnesses may cease to exist in the
future. According to a WHO report on Global Burden of Disease [12], uni-polar
depressive disorders are the number one cause of burden of disease in developed
countries. In 2030, the same thing is expected to be true for the entire World.

Table 12.1 Several mental illnesses, symptoms and target population

Group of Mental Illnesses	Example	Symptoms	Target population
Mood Disorders	Major depression	Lack of energy, sleep, and interests Suicidal ideations	Young adults, adults, and geriatric population
	Bi-polar or manic-depressive disorder	Manic phase followed by depressive phase	Young adults, adults, and geriatric population
Cognitive Disorders	Alzheimer	Severe forgetfulness	Older adults
Personality disorders	Obsessive-Compulsive	Distress in job and family situations	Young adults and adults
Schizophrenia	Paranoid Type Schizophrenia	Hallucinations Delusions	Young adults, adults, and geriatric population
Anxiety Disorders	Panic disorder	Panic attacks Excessive worrying	Young adults, adults, and geriatric population
	Post Traumatic Stress Disorder	Excessive alertness Lack of sleep	All age groups
Eating Disorder	Anorexia Nervosa	Loss of weight Abnormal heart rhythm	Primarily young and adult women
Developmental disorder	Attention deficit disorder	Inability to focus	Primarily children

12.1.1 Problems in Mental Health Services

The current situation is also exacerbated due to society's distorted perception of
mental illnesses, shortage and training of healthcare workers, access to easy-
prescription where some people claim anything to get a certain medication and
any government benefits such as disability, confusion among the role of psychiatrists and psychologists, and media playing the role of psychiatrist. For example,

psychologists can provide a range of mental health services including psychotherapy, however, psychiatrists could do these and also write prescriptions for medications. In addition, some healthcare professionals, seemingly trying to avoid confrontation with patients, prefer writing controlled substances for years even when patients do not need them or when newer non-addictive options become available. A related and more recent problem includes the abuse of prescription drugs for academic performance enhancement in some countries including the US. This involves some parents coercing healthcare professionals to write stimulants for kids, who do not need these medically but take these anyway for improving academic performance. This may help parents, kids, healthcare professionals, and drug companies at the expense of federal government, taxpayers, and insurance companies. These stimulants, while not necessarily addictive in the prescribed amount, could be addictive if abused in higher dosages. The brain chemistry of kids could change over time, potentially resulting in the incidence of one or more severe mental illnesses.

12.1.2 Mental Status Examination

Overall, there is a large number of overlapping and difficult to understand illnesses and only qualified healthcare professionals can make certain determinations. These diagnoses are made by comprehensive evaluation including history of present illness, past psychiatric and medical history, substance abuse history, family and personal-social history, review of major health systems, and mental status examination usually in the first appointment with a healthcare professional, although MSE can be repeated. In general, mental status examination includes evaluating the following factors:

- The level of consciousness (alert, drowsy)
- Attitude (negative, apprehensive, positive)
- Behavior (co-operative, uncooperative, defensive, hostile)
- Cognition (memory registration and recall)
- Mood (depressed, labile, anxious)
- Affect (sad, happy, dysphoric)
- Range of emotions (constricted, flat, blunted)
- Speech (latency, volume, goal-directed)
- Motor (psychomotor retardation, agitation)
- Thought content (suicidal, hallucinations, phobias, delusions)
- Thought processes (linear, flight of ideas, tangential)
- Insight (recognition of problem)
- Judgment (problem solving, impulse control, IQ, abstract thinking)

It is possible that a patient may suffer from multiple mental illnesses at the same time and such determination is possible using MSE and further psychological testing.

12.1.3 Symptoms and Hospitalization

Some of the mental illnesses show clear and strong symptoms, such as Major Depression which involves overwhelming sadness or despair, difficulty sleeping, lack of interests in usual activities for more than 14 days. However, some variations of depression are more subtle and patients may not be aware of their presence such as Dysthymia, a low-grade depression with symptoms lasting over years.

Patients with mental illnesses could be monitored and treated in outpatient facilities for depression and mood-disorders; anxiety and panic attacks; substance abuse; post traumatic stress disorder and some loss of functioning. However, in some cases patients may need to be kept in a hospital, voluntarily or involuntarily. It should be noted that some hospitals only allow voluntary hospitalization and may transfer serious patients, once medically stable, to other hospitals with involuntary medical facilities. The symptoms and signs that require immediate physician attention or hospitalization are

- suicidal ideation, with or without intent or plan
- homicidal ideation, with or without intent or plan
- unstable or out of control due to mania, agitation, acute psychosis
- dementia with severe behavioral problems (such as resisting care, wandering away, at risk for harm to self or others)
- dementia with psychotic symptoms
- delirious patient if medically stable
- serious withdrawal for drugs
- rapid, sudden and severe deterioration of functioning

In addition to these, patients living in assisted living and nursing homes may require such attention and/or hospitalization, if one or more of the followings occur

- difficult, demanding, and loud patient causing disruption
- patient threatening to leave against medical advice
- repetitive disruptive behaviors and agitating and dangerous to other residents

There is a need to monitor behavior and other symptoms to provide continued care and recovery. Just like physical illnesses, people with mental illnesses can be treated and monitored for a range of conditions and provided medical care as necessary.

12.2 Challenges in Mental Health Monitoring

There are many challenges in mental health monitoring. These include monitoring of behavior, which is much more complex and dynamic than physical symptoms, and requires new methods and techniques to measure several parameters and evaluate behavioral conditions including suicidal and homicidal ideations.

There is much more stigma attached with mental health, this could make patients and their relatives much more sensitive to privacy and HIPAA rules. The need to protect privacy is enormous and mental health monitoring systems should protect patient privacy and any information collected in the monitoring process just like any other HIPAA compliant monitoring. Although in many cases, patients may want to be monitored based on the advice of healthcare professionals, but in many cases, the patients and family members would have to be convinced to allow monitoring of one or more mental health conditions. They must be able to see the clear benefits of such monitoring and any improvements to the overall mental health of the monitored patients. Several stakeholders including healthcare professionals and insurance companies may have to be involved in creating very supportive and convincing environment for family members and patients to agree to such monitoring. In some extreme cases, including when a patient does not want to stay in the hospitals and leaves against the medical advice, laws may have to be clarified/modified to require mental health monitoring of such patient.

There is also a higher chance of addiction to prescription drugs, controlled substances, and even illegal drugs. Thus, mental health monitoring should include monitoring for addiction. Patients with mental health problems are likely to have cognitive decline or problems, some in younger patients and some in older patients due to aging, which makes their day-to-day life much more difficult. This also requires that monitoring systems and patients' surroundings offer them much more support in helping their day to day life. Additional challenges include possible paranoia with technology, diversity of patients such as child and adolescents, adult, and geriatric patients. Although some patients could stay in assisted living and/or nursing homes, some patients need the institutional care such as state hospitals or a private hospital-psychiatry unit. With a large number of older patients worldwide, the number of people needing care for dementia, including Alzheimer's, is rapidly increasing. Since most of the monitoring is voluntary, work is needed to evaluate the patient adherence to mental health monitoring.

A new field of wireless psychiatry, or a way to address many problems using wireless technologies, is emerging. This will include comprehensive monitoring of patients for symptoms, behavior, and medication compliance. The monitoring for behavior includes suicidal and homicidal behavior in nursing homes, assisted living, home care, hospitals, and in society-at large. The monitoring for medication compliance could be facilitated by designing and employing smart-pill-containers, which dispense medications and also generate alerts for physicians for compliance and/or abuse. This also includes monitoring for related physical conditions such as sleep patterns, weight loss as part of depression and suicidal behavior, and weight gain due to inactivity and certain medications. Also, the support for location tracking of patients, services, hospitals, and healthcare services; remote help for emergencies, hospitalization, police, ambulance; telemedicine and tele-therapy; cognitive assistance in the form of who they are, where they are, what they are, and with whom they are; and use of context-awareness. In addition, all patient information will be made available to physicians before their appointment with the patients. This will allow patients with cognitive problems to help describe their problems while the ones with imaginary problems will be checked with their monitored information.

12.3 Examples of MHM

With an increasing number of people worldwide suffering from one or more mental illnesses, including anxiety and depressive disorders to Alzheimer and other dementias. The incidence has been increasing in all segments of the population and is particularly high in the elder population. Wireless patient monitoring systems can be designed for monitoring patient's conditions. This will allow that patient's mental health can be monitored from a distance, especially when a patient cannot frequently or routinely travel to a physician's office or a hospital. The basic idea is the same as in WHM of other illnesses and that is to monitor certain conditions and if one or more of these seem to be severe enough, then either the patient is hospitalized and/or some treatment is changed/offered. The monitoring could include monitoring of vital signs and activity levels. This can be supplemented with subjective symptoms from the patient and objective symptoms from the family members. This may require some training to the family members on what to observe and report to healthcare professionals. It should be noted that a combination of symptoms and problems reported by a patient and family members would lead to a more accurate description of what is happening than by just listening to the subjective symptoms from the patient only. Also, a range of daily activities can be included along with medication adherence or whether the person has been taking the prescribed medicines regularly or not. The symptoms that could be reported over a wireless device include sleep, appetite, energy level, apprehension, lack of interest, psychosis, and, suicidal and/or homicidal behaviors (Figure 12.1). If a patient's picture or video can be taken and transmitted over the network to a healthcare professional, then one of several conditions can also be checked. These could include anxiety symptoms, pain-score, level of depression, and other general symptoms. In practice, more work can be done in transmitting only the medically needed part of the picture or video and filtering out rest of the picture to allow for immediate transmission and viewing of the picture during a session. This will also reduce the cognitive overload of the healthcare professionals. The other possibility is to transmit a patient's picture or video periodically for healthcare professionals to see longer-term view and any changes in the patient's conditions. Any discrepancy observed in the information provided by a patient and/or family members and the information obtained by wireless monitoring can be used to check the authenticity of symptoms, if faked to obtain secondary gains. These could include disability benefits; excuse for not returning to work, school, or performing house duties.

To protect the patient's privacy and to avoid any misuse of the information, the monitoring system should be highly secure and the access to such information should be limited only to those authorized by the patient or his/her legal guardians.

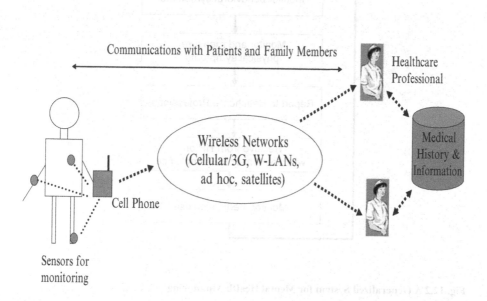

Communications with Patients and Family Members

Healthcare Professional

Wireless Networks (Cellular/3G, W-LANs, ad hoc, satellites)

Cell Phone

Medical History & Information

Sensors for monitoring

Fig 12.1 Mental Health Monitoring

Next, we derive a generalized system for mental health monitoring. This system can be used for monitoring a large number of mental illnesses. This works by finding out what are the specific symptoms that need to be monitored. Then the symptoms are broken into behavioral and physical symptoms. These symptoms can be received from multiple sources such as patients, family members and/or sensors. These are then processed based on specified thresholds and then reported to the designated healthcare professional. The healthcare professional will inform the system on what else needs to be monitored, such as patient's physical activity, compliance to medication, and attendance at group meetings if suggested. This system can be used for monitoring of several specific conditions discussed in the next few subsections.

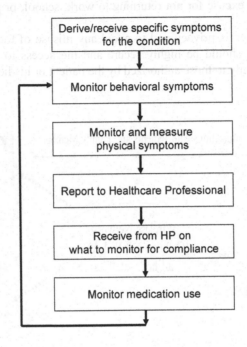

Fig. 12.2 A Generalized System for Mental Health Monitoring

12.3.1 Alzheimer Monitoring

Alzheimer's dementia can be monitored and diagnosed from a distance by finding out if the patient is having confusion, forgetfulness and/or dis-orientation and is showing signs of sun-downing or a set of strange behaviors after sunset. This could include agitation, wandering, restlessness, panic, psychosis, and depression. The patient may report some subjective symptoms, based on his/her memory and behavioral conditions. The family could report more details on nutrition, hypogly-cemia and include other daily observations. The level of agitation could be scored based on the patient's actions, which could involve simple screaming to full-blown physical fight/abuse to others. A video or picture of patient's behavior may also help in monitoring/diagnosing using one of several different systems of scoring symptoms and facial expressions of the patient. These could also be applied to many other mental illnesses such as chronic pain, depression, and bipolar disorders. In practice, the patient may see the physician occasionally and remain under monitoring between possible visits. In some extreme cases, where travel is extremely limited due to a variety of reasons, the monitoring system can facilitate a meeting among physician, patient and family members.

About 20% of elderly use computers and decline in their cognitive functions can be monitored by their interactions with computers [13]. More specifically, the work involves unobtrusively monitoring of computer interactions to detect changes in cognitive performance. The algorithms for inferring a user's cognitive performance using monitoring data from computer games and psychomotor measurements associated with keyboard entry and mouse movement are developed [13]. The inferences are then used to classify significant performance changes [13]. The work is applicable to early detection of cognitive decline and thus may support the use of newer medications available for the early treatment of dementia.

12.3.2 Post Traumatic Stress Disorder Monitoring

PTSD represents an immediate or delayed response to one or more traumatic events such as war, abuse, natural and man-made disasters. The responses include an intense fear, helplessness and horror. The PTSD symptoms are increased vigilance or alertness and difficulty sleeping. It usually develops within 3 months of the trauma but can also begin years later [2].

The treatment normally includes medications and psychotherapy to teach patients how to handle anxiety-provoking situations. Also, participation in a support group with people who have gone through similar experiences has been shown to be very helpful.

The wireless health monitoring of PTSD could include people that have experienced trauma recently, such as those returning from a war, and people who have been through trauma or abuse. In some cases, preventative monitoring, useful for people returning home from war, could be used to observe if someone is beginning to show signs of PTSD and treat, if necessary, before it becomes severe.

The PTSD monitoring can include activity monitoring, sleep monitoring, and ECG in detecting PTSD. A range of wearable and environmental sensors can be used for the monitoring. The sleep monitoring can be implemented by adding pressure and/or thermal sensors to the patient's bed. ECG signals can be monitored by using wearable body sensors and/or sensors in bed, bathroom, and other objects the patient may come in contact [3]. The sleep monitoring can assist in detecting the level of sleep the person is enjoying. The ECG may show palpitations that occur in people suffering from PTSD. Thus, WHM can be used in detecting as well as long-term monitoring of PTSD symptoms.

The wireless infrastructure of patient monitoring may also enable patients, in close proximity and have agreed to a group, to form one or more support groups. The conversations and discussion of the group could be recorded and sent securely to a healthcare professional to evaluate the effectiveness of the group. Once evaluated, such recordings should be deleted to avoid misuse or privacy violations. In some cases, some changes in the group may be needed to provide the patients with most needed help. If the symptoms worsen, the patients may have to be hospitalized and/or given medications to relieve symptoms of sleeplessness.

12.3.3 Monitoring of Obsessive Compulsive Disorder (OCD)

OCD is a mental disorder in the general class of anxiety disorders, characterized by mild to severe persistent, intrusive thoughts, images, or impulses (obsessions) that a person tries to compensate for with repetitive actions (compulsions). When the symptoms worsen, the patient may require medications, behavioral therapy, or hospitalization. Both subjective and objective reports, including any major stress factors, from the patient and family members, respectively, can be used in determining the presence or severity of the OCD. The monitoring of OCD could involve monitoring of user activities and determination if these activities are repetitive. For each activity a user has been involved for some time, the WPM system can keep a counter and if that exceeds a threshold (set by healthcare professionals), a message can be sent to a healthcare professional. The monitoring system may develop a list of activities the patient normally undertakes and creates a frequency and duration counters for each activity. Data mining techniques can be used to produce the patient's behavioral pattern and decide normal or abnormal behavior. Most certainly, more work is needed in designing, developing, implementing and testing wireless monitoring systems for OCD.

12.3.4 Monitoring of Panic Disorder

This illness causes repeated, frequent and unexpected panic attacks, which are sudden and overwhelming episodes of anxiety in which the person feels out of control and threatened with imminent harm [2]. The panic disorder must have three components: the presence of panic attacks, the unexpectedness of panic attacks, and anxiety over future attacks lasting more than a month [2]. Some of the most common physical symptoms are chest pain, shortness of breath, heart palpitations, sweating, and agitations. Wireless monitoring system, more likely to be of wearable type, could measure many of these symptoms over a month and thus could help determine the presence or absence of panic disorder. Although the monitoring system here would be programmed to store patient's symptoms for later analysis, it should still generate alarms for healthcare professionals in case of severe symptoms which may indicate other illness such as cardiovascular. Any prior history of other illnesses, especially the ones with overlapping or similar symptoms, should be programmed as context information to the monitoring system.

12.3.5 Monitoring of Eating Disorders

Another very helpful monitoring could involve wireless monitoring of people suffering from weight and body-image disorders including anorexia nervosa, bulimia, and pica or abnormal craving for inorganic substances.

Anorexia nervosa is a mental illness in which a person refuses to maintain normal body weight, is extremely afraid of gaining weight and has a distorted image of his or her body [2]. People suffering from this illness restrict both the quantity and type of food they eat and are known to purge food out of their bodies. The disease primarily affects women in their teens but could continue in adulthood and is known to be accompanied by other mental illnesses [2]. Bulimia is another mental illness characterized by recurrent episodes of binge eating and extreme countermeasures to reduce the impact of food, often by self-induced vomiting [2]. To be characterized as Bulimia, the episodes must occur at least twice a week for three months.

The episodes of binge eating may be detected by wireless sensors placed around people's neck to measure the amount and frequency of swallowing. Another set of sensors could be developed to monitor purging including vomiting and use of laxatives to eliminate food ingested. If algorithms/methods could be devised that somehow can differentiate between normal and self-induced vomiting, such as by detecting the presence of fingers in the mouth before vomiting, then it may be quite possible to monitor eating disorders form a distance over a long-term period.

Out of many known physical symptoms, some are measurable and could include measuring symptoms of depression, anxiety, substance abuse, excessive exercise, and more critically weight loss. Additionally, abnormal heart rhythm could be monitored. If detected, long-term monitoring can also be combined with psychotherapy and counseling on eating balanced diet to maintain normal weight.

12.3.6 Monitoring of Autistic Behavior

Autism is a nervous system disorder that begins in early childhood and is characterized by impaired social interaction, problems with communication and imagination, and unusual or limited activities or interests [2]. Majority of people suffering have mental retardation and repetitive, unusual, aggressive and self-injurious behavior. Educational and behavioral interventions can help developing social skills and medications to moderate aggressive behavior.

Wireless monitoring systems can be designed to monitor behavior and social interactions, such as by measuring the frequency and amount of time a person under monitoring stays in close proximity of another person and by recording the number/type of words exchanged. This could be facilitated by use of wearable computing system that include camera to record some of these actions and interactions. This may then be processed by algorithms/schemes to derive the level of social interactions/skills and behavior. Additionally, sensors can detect leg, hand and body movements along with words in detecting presence/absence of violent and aggressive behavior. Certainly much more work is needed in developing a wireless monitoring system for autism and other pervasive developmental disorders.

12.4 Monitoring of Medication Compliance and Addiction

With the number of US prescriptions filled in 2006 reaching to 2.4 billion, the cost for prescription medications is a major component of healthcare expenses. It would be acceptable if all the medications prescribed and bought were used for intended purposes. However, the use of medications ranges from no-use (about one third), infrequent use (about one third), and overuse to abuse (about one third). The non-adherence to medications leads to more than 125,000 deaths in the US and more than $90 billion in additional hospitalization and procedures every year [4]. Additionally, people who miss their doses are three times more likely to see doctors again, resulting in further increase in healthcare expenses. According to NIH [5], about 20% of the people in the US have used prescription drugs for non-medical reasons, also known as prescription drug abuse. Some of the prescription medications, especially narcotics; sedatives, hypnotics, and anxiolytics; and stimulants, could lead to addiction, which in turn requires detoxification and rehabilitation. This further increases the cost of healthcare including the need for additional medications.

To address the above challenges, there has been some work towards increasing the medication adherence. Most interventions for adherence fall into three categories:
1. Educational: Information conveyed verbally and in writing to patients
2. Behavioral: reminders, contracts, drug packaging
3. Affective: Counseling, home visits, and family support.

These interventions have helped improving the adherence, but it is still not satisfactory. The key challenges in medication adherence are (a) some patients not getting their prescriptions filled, (b) some of the patients who are getting their prescription filled are using it infrequently or discontinuing at will and (c) some are using "catch-up" to take an overdose for compensating missed dosages. In prescription drug abuse, (a) some patients are doing intentional overdose and (b) some are diverting (buying/selling) prescription of controlled substances or having multiple prescriptions for the same condition by "doctor shopping" for addiction problems. Healthcare Information Technologies (HIT), especially wireless and mobile technologies, can address some of these challenges. Even a small improvement in the adherence to medications can save millions of precious healthcare dollars everyday. To identify and use these technologies, there is a need to study and model these challenges and technologies and then to derive and design technology-based solutions for enhancing adherence to as well as limiting abuse of prescription medications.

12.4.1 Medication Management & Potential Problems

Medication management has been done by patients and family members for long time in several different ad hoc ways. These could range from using sticky notes, organization of medicines, and reminders. There has been some work on studying how elders manage their medications currently and how such methods may be incorporated in future assistive technologies for medication adherence [15]. More specifically, an ethnographic study has identified that some elders devise medication management systems using the spatial features of their homes, their daily routines, and how and when they visit certain places in their house to help remember them to take their medications [15]. The study also presents several principles for the design of assistive technologies for future personalized medication systems.

Recently, information technologies have been proposed for supporting medication management, where patients can be reminded to take their medications at certain times. The implementation is usually a pill container (Figure 12.3) with alarms that go-off at certain times and the pill container remembers how many times it has been opened and closed. Such reminders along with reminders from family members and healthcare professionals could increase the compliance to medications, especially for patients with cognitive and/or physical disabilities. An example is Magic Medicine Cabinet (MMC), designed to enable reminding and ensuring to take the right medicine, measure vital signs, inform about conditions, and interact with healthcare professionals [14]. The MMC uses both voice and embedded display for reminders to a patient. It employs Internet connectivity, face recognition, RFID-based smart labels, vital sign monitors, touch-sensitive screen, and voice synthesis for reminders [14]. Another example is smart medicine cabinet designed to support mobile and young patients with chronic diseases [16]. The features include use of reminders, query for contents (medications), expiry date detection, and alarms for product recalls. The system utilizes both passive and active RFID tags to monitor medication boxes and to communicate with a cell phone, respectively.

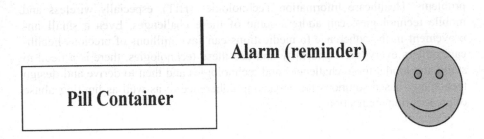

Fig. 12.3 Basic Medication Management System

In addition to an increased level of adherence, medication management should also lead to reduction in potential abuse for controlled substances such as narcotic painkillers, sedatives, and stimulants. One way to enhance adherence to medications and also to reduce misuse and abuse is to employ wireless technologies where a medication is only allowed to be dispensed with *certain doses* at *a certain number of times a day* to *certain people*. This smart medication management system (SMMS) can also keep track of the time and the number of times/day a certain medication was taken. Also, for future modifications, it can keep track of how many times a patient attempted to open the medication system without success. Physicians can check/communicate with the SMMS on medication adherence and/or abuse before renewing the prescriptions. For consistent abuse, the first few violations can be notified to physicians and then to law enforcement and insurance companies. SMMS can't stop drug abuse but it can certainly reduce it. Patients can give the dispensed medicine to someone else but only one dose at a time, which makes it less profitable than selling the whole prescription.

Physicians can periodically check if their patients are abusing drugs. For example, a healthcare professional may need to check 1000+ patients. This can be done serially or just on a probabilistic basis such as creating list of all the patients on controlled substances and having an appointment next week. Then the physician can limit future prescription to few days at a time as oppose to 30-day supplies of medications. In addition, all patient information will be made available to healthcare professionals by SMMS before their appointment with the patients. This will allow patients with cognitive problems to help describe their problems while the ones with imaginary problems will be checked with their monitored information.

There are many *advantages* of such medication systems. These include improvement in adherence level resulting in better utilization of already occurred healthcare expenses, reduced number of hospitalizations, and better health outcomes including reduced morbidity, reduced mortality, and improved quality of life. Also, in some cases, it will lead to some reduction of medication abuse due to the inability in getting multiple doses at a time and the ability of the medication system in monitoring and recording patient's medication usage behavior, including the number of times a "forced entry" was attempted. If the patient has "diverted" a prescription or employed "doctor-shopping", the medication system can also check for the presence of multiple similar prescriptions in its vicinity. Overall, the medication management system could lead to reduction in both existing healthcare cost of prescriptions and future healthcare cost of treating patients for a lack of health improvement and/or addiction.

There are several potential *disadvantages* of medication systems. These include potential for reduced adherence if the medication management system is very restrictive and inflexible, the total cost of medication management system including the hardware and software cost, and, difficulty in use with changes in patient's or healthcare professional's schedule and travel. Also, a major challenge is obtaining patient's consent for monitoring of his/her medication usage. Also, such system may fail or could become inaccessible for some reason, resulting in a patient missing an important dose. To avoid this, medication systems should support switching to a manual mode of operation in case of failure or other problems. Other backup measures may also be in order to help patient comply with medications.

12.4.2 Smart Medication Management System

A range of information technologies, which can be utilized to support medication management system, must be considered. Among others, it will include the use of several networks that can be formed among SMMS, radio-enabled devices and sensors for enhancing the quality and reliability of adherence monitoring. Such wireless networks will also allow the SMMS to interface with EMR and m-prescriptions for improving the patient safety, and monitoring with the compliance with prescriptions using Bluetooth and sensors, and notifications to physicians for one or more such problems.

A range of SMMS implementations could be developed in the future for different applications and environment. These could include purely medication *support* systems, supporting reminders and alarms to patients, and measurement of the adherence to medications, to highly active *monitoring* systems that would also monitor and limit any abuse by restricting access, enforcing authorization, and checking for similar drugs in the patient's vicinity.

A high-level view of how SMMS would operate and interface with patients, healthcare professionals, and networks is shown in Figure 12.4. The SMMS would be programmable and controllable remotely and interact with healthcare professionals and patients. We envision that both drug adherence and drug abuse can be monitored as and when needed. In majority of cases, only drug adherence monitoring may be required, while in some cases involving patients with a history or

controlled substances, drug abuse monitoring will also be enabled. The SMMS
will be flexible, easy-to-use, customized to patient's abilities, programmable, and
reusable to reduce the overall cost. To ensure that the patient has consumed the
dispensed medication, swallowing detection sensors could be employed. The sensors
will communicate with the SMMS any sensed parameters to indicate that the
patient has swallowed the medication. If the sensors could also verify that a specific
medication has been swallowed by the patient, and not some candy, it will
improve the accuracy of medication monitoring. Certainly there are ways to outsmart SMMS or sensors, however, these can determine the level of adherence a
patient is showing.

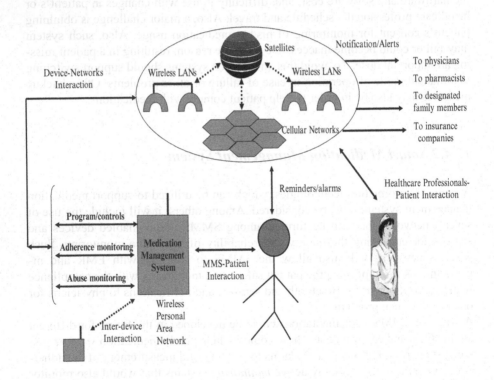

Fig. 12.4 SMMS and Interworking with Patients and Healthcare Professionals

List of SMMS Functions:

1. Find out information on medications and authorized persons (the number of
   doses per day, persons authorized)

2. Find out which type of monitoring has to be turned-on and for how long
3. When and how (voice, video monitor, display board) to generate alarms as reminder to patients
4. List of people who needs to be notified if certain undesirable events occur
5. Manage network connectivity to the list of people (and if not possible for some time, locally record the information and upload as soon as network connectivity becomes possible again)
6. Manage the dispensing of medications by opening a small outlet of a pill size (certain duration when the outlet is opened, check medications just before the outlet is open and just after the outlet is closed again, send alarms to necessary people if the difference between the two is more than the allowed dosage)
7. Process any notifications to and from a list of places/people.
8. Support personalization for patients and adaptive operation of SMMS
9. If "abuse" monitoring is on
Check for similar drugs in the vicinity for the patient
Keep track of how many times pressure has been applied to "forced" open the pill bottle
Send notifications to people on the list for undesirable events
10. If patient-travel-support = Yes
Allow more flexibility
Still record the usage and send to the list when connected to networks again (have an ability to connect to available networks as quickly as possible)

12.4.3 Evaluation of SMMS

As there has been little work on medication systems, no metrics are available for evaluation. The following three metrics can be used for measuring the effectiveness of SMMS for medication adherence:

- The level of compliance (fraction of times the correct dose is taken)
- The number of unsuccessful attempts as a measure of abuse reduction by SMMS
- The network traffic per monitored patient

Several different adherence models could be employed covering a range of patients, from teenagers to geriatric patients, in youth care, home care, assisted living and nursing homes to validate SMMS. The adherence models will include complete-self-care, assisted-care, and complete-dependent-care to cover scenarios of levels of control over consumption of prescription medications. These models will provide a realistic assessment of effectiveness of the SMMS (Figure 12.5). In addition to validation and evaluation, daily, weekly and long-term adherence can be measured to provide more detailed insight in the medication usage patterns. The number of messages over wireless networks can also be measured to study potential overhead and complexity, and could also be employed in continued SMMS design improvements. More work can also be done on when and how the "monitoring" part of SMMS should be utilized and who should be notified for non-adherence and its impact on SMMS complexity and network traffic. More work is also needed in enhancing or supporting the level of personalization in SMMS.

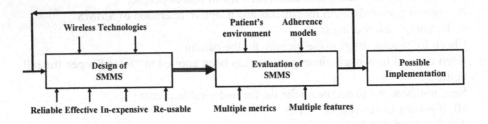

Fig. 12.5 Evaluation of SMMS using Several Models

The possible extensions of MMS and additional capabilities are potentially limitless as it

1. Could be combined with health monitoring systems (such as vital signs, sleep patterns, weight loss) and behavior monitoring systems (depression, suicidal and homicidal behavior: in nursing homes, assisted living, home care, hospitals, and in society-at large)
2. Could be combined with location tracking (patients, services, hospitals, and healthcare services) and remote-help systems (emergencies, hospitalization, police, ambulance)
3. Can be expanded to provide cognitive assistance to patients (who they are, where they are, and what they are, where they are, and with whom they are)

12.5 Disability Monitoring and Verification

According to National Health Interview Survey, it has been estimated that 19.4 million medically treatable injuries occur in the working-age adults in the United States. Among employed persons, 38% of injuries occurred at work, and among employed men aged 55–64 years, 49% of injuries occurred at work [6]. In the workplace, the number of injuries is estimated to be 5.5 million/year [6]. According to the National Safety Council, the average cost of wage and productivity losses, medical expenses, and administrative expenses for a disabling injury at work is $38,000 [7]. According to OSHA, the injury and illness rate has been declining and in 2005, it reached to 4.6/year per 100 workers for serious injuries [8]. According to the Workplace Safety Index the three leading causes of serious on-the-job injuries are Overexertion, Falls on Same Level and Bodily Reaction and result in about $23 billion a year or $450 million a week [9].

After the injury has occurred, many patients are hospitalized and provided necessary healthcare services. Once discharged, most get back to work with one or more restrictions, however many workers claim to be have some form of disability. Some of the disabilities are clearly obvious, while others are subject to interpretation. These patients then file workers' compensation claims and the employers' insurance company starts processing the claims. Although most of such claims are genuine, these claims have to go through serious scrutiny thus affecting both genuine and fraudulent cases.

About 60% of serious injuries involve PPD (Permanent Partial Disability) and averages about $61,000 [10]. In addition, these claims could also become eligible for federal government benefits, such as social security disability income. Many of these injuries may also lead to emotional and psychological problems, including depression, anxiety, and panic attacks, which are subjectively reported and objectively diagnosed by physicians during the clinic visit using a set of standardized interviews and evaluation. However, no longitudinal assessment of their conditions before and after the clinic visit can be made. There is some anecdotal evidence of patients feigning symptoms to receive physician's letter stating their "disability". One of the major causes of such disability is the "presence" of chronic pain, leading to potential for receiving opioids analgesic agents despite of newer treatments such as epidural block, nerve root ablation, discectomy, spinal cord stimulators, and, TENS (Transcutaneous Electrical Nerve Stimulator) unit. The data on such fraud is hard to find, but has been estimated from 3% to 20% depending on the source. This could lead to an estimated $4-22 billion/year in fraudulent disability claims.

This presents the following challenges:
1. The genuine cases are delayed before their rightful compensation is paid, thus affecting the lives of a large number of such patients.
2. The fraudulent cases may not receive as much scrutiny as these deserve and thus may not be detected, leading to potentially hundreds of millions

paid to such claims and affecting the total cost, including the cost of healthcare services and an increased insurance premium for employers.

3. Insurance companies may spend a considerable amount of resources in processing, verifying, and detecting all claims, resulting in a significant cost increase in doing their business, thus also potentially limiting the amount of award to genuine patients.

So there is a need to design and develop a system that can monitor patients conditions for a certain time, help genuine patients get their rightful payment quickly, and reduce frauds related to feigned injuries. We envision that such system will create some evidence, which can be used in determining a variety of disability claims. Such system will not replace the existing claims processing and litigations, but could assist in creating some evidence, which in conjunction with other information, can assist decision making in disability verification.

A wireless-monitoring based assistant can be designed and developed to monitor the condition of a patient, who has filed a claim for workers compensation. The WPM-assistant will monitor multiple vital signs and other biomedical parameters, depending on the claimed disability, and record these for throughout the monitoring duration determined and agreed upon by all sides. The purpose of this assistant is to create an additional set of evidence that can be considered in determining whether a claimed condition exists or not. This assistant could help those that are really hurt and really deserve the claimed compensation. It would also help insurance companies and employers in detecting fraudulent claims.

12.5.1 WPM Disability-Assistant

The WPM disability-assistant will monitor multiple conditions, personalized to the patient, and will detect and record any such conditions for certain duration. This will involve voluntary placement and the refusal to place on his/her body cannot be perceived as a presence of guilt or fraud. The WPM disability-assistant is highly personalized for the patient by programming it to the past medical history, claimed disability conditions, and specific medical knowledge. The recording of patient's vital signs and other information over the duration specified and agreed upon all parties. It could have alarms for certain conditions using context-aware actions, such as if a patient has claimed to have serious back injury and is lifting heavy objects, the monitoring assistant will detect changes in vital signs along with movements in a set of muscles (Figure 12.6). This is not a complete disability verification system, but is designed to be an assistive tool to create some evidence to be used in determining the claimed disability.

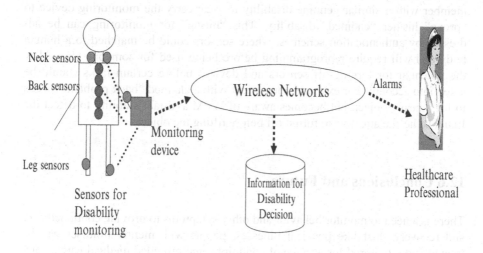

Fig. 12.6 The Design and Operation of Disability Assistant

12.5.2 Implementation Challenges

There are several challenges in using WPM disability-assistant. These include a loss of patient privacy, which has to be carefully considered against any future benefits derived from the desired disability status. Some patients may have a fear of monitoring especially those suffering from emotional and psychological problems and may be uncomfortable with a continuous monitoring system that could generate information against their claims. The information generated by WPM assistant should only be used in deciding disability status and there should be no potential for self-incrimination (5th amendment to the constitution and a basic right in the US). The patients can refuse the use of a monitoring agent anytime before or during the specified duration. The ownership of collected information should be decided to avoid any future problems for the monitored patients. The possibilities are deletion of such information about the disability case is decided or allowing the involved patients to have the ownership rights on such information.

The assistant should be matched to the physical strength and capability of patients and could be wearable vs portable. There may be reliability challenges, where the sensors may not work as intended and hurt the chances of honest patients.

There is still some potential for continued fraud even with the use of WPM assistant. For example, the patient could find someone living nearby or even a family member with a similar genuine disability to wear/carry the monitoring device to "prove" his/her "claimed" disability. This "hiring" for monitoring can be addressed by authentication schemes, where sensors could be matched to a human body and will require reprogramming before being used for someone else. Also, the potential for turning-off sensors and devices before certain tasks should be taken into account. For example, the patient with a claimed "back problem" needs to lift a heavy object, but becomes aware of WPM assistant's ability to detect the fraud, so he/she attempts to turn it off before lifting the object.

12.6 Conclusions and Future

There is a need to monitor behavior and other symptoms to provide continued care and recovery. Just like physical illnesses, people with mental illnesses can be treated and monitored for a range of conditions and provided medical care as and when necessary. There are many challenges in mental health monitoring. These include monitoring of behavior, which requires new methods and techniques to measure several parameters and evaluate behavioral conditions including suicidal and homicidal ideations. Mental health monitoring should include monitoring for addiction. The patients with mental health are likely to have cognitive decline or problems, which makes their day to day life much more difficult. This also requires that monitoring systems offer them much more support in helping their day-to-day life.

A new field of wireless psychiatry, or a way to address many behavioral and mental illnesses using wireless technologies, is emerging. This includes comprehensive monitoring of patients for symptoms, behavior, and medication compliance. The monitoring for behavior includes in general behavior in nursing homes, assisted living, home care, hospitals, and in society-at large. The monitoring for medication compliance could be facilitated by designing and employing smart-pill-containers, which dispense medications and also generate alerts for physicians for compliance and/or abuse. This also includes monitoring for related physical conditions such as sleep patterns, weight loss as part of depression, and weight gain due to inactivity and certain medications.

For future work, there is a need to design new methods, techniques and algorithms to match a variety of sensed parameters and signs into behavioral patterns, episodes and mental illnesses. The use of context can be very helpful to identify specific illness out of several possible choices. Many new mental health monitoring applications can be designed to monitor conditions identified in this chapter. Additional work can also be done in addressing the usability challenges of wireless and wearable technologies for a diversity of mental health patients ranging from children to adults to older people. There is also some need for the design of autonomous systems that are also free from patient's destructive actions taken under episodes of mental illness. Mental health monitoring systems should also be optimized and personalized to the patient and work reliably over the entire duration of monitoring for providing the best care possible.

Questions:

1. What can be done to stop kids from taking stimulants for improving academic performance?
2. Describe a mental health condition (not discussed in the text) which could be monitored by wireless networks. List symptoms that you would like to monitor and show how.
3. Panic attacks could also occur as a result of substance intoxication or substance withdrawal. How would you monitor someone who is abusing substances (drugs, alcohol)?
4. Think of several ways in which a patient could outsmart the SMMS. Think of changes that can be made in the SMMS to avoid these problems.
5. Describe how disability assistant work? What is your opinion on possible deployment of such systems for disability monitoring?
6. How to ensure that disability assistant would work properly throughout the duration of monitoring?

References:
[1] Mental Health: A Report of the Surgeon General, 1999 Website: http://mentalhealth.samhsa.gov/features/surgeongeneralreport/chapter1/sec1.asp#approach (accessed on July 21, 2008)
[2] AMA Concise Medical Encyclopedia (Medical Editor: Martin Lipsky), Random House Reference, 2006
[3] Ogawa M, Togawa T (2003) The concept of home health monitoring. In Proc. of 5th International Workshop on Enterprise Networking and Computing in Healthcare Industry (Healthcom)
[4] Mpill website: http://www.m-pill.com/index.php?browse=compliance (accessed on July 21, 2008)
[5] NIH website for prescription drug abuse: http://www.nlm.nih.gov/medlineplus/prescriptiondrugabuse.html (accessed on July 21, 2008)
[6] Smith G. et. al. (2005) Injuries at work in the us adult population: contributions to the total injury burden. American Journal of Public Health, 95(7):1213-1219, July
[7] National Safety Council's website (http://www.nsc.org/lrs/statinfo/estcost.htm)
[8] The US Dept. of Labor, Occupational Safety and Health Administration, http://www.osha.gov/dep/enforcement/enforcement_results_06.html
[9] The website for Workplace Safety Index http://www.hss.energy.gov/HealthSafety/WSHA/vpp/articles/injuries.html
[10] The website for NCPA: http://www.ncpa.org/pub/st/st287/st287b.html

[11] Varshney U (2007) Pervasive healthcare and wireless patient monitoring. ACM/Springer Journal on Mobile Networks and Applications (MONET), 12(2-3):113-127, March

[12] WHO 2004 Report on Global Burden of Disease: http://www.who.int/healthinfo/global_burden_disease/GBD_report_2004update_part4.pdf

[13] Jimison H, Pavel M, McKanna J, Pavel J (2004) Unobtrusive monitoring of computer interactions to detect cognitive status in elders. IEEE Trans. Inf. Technol. Biomed. 8(3): 248-252, Sept.

[14] Wan D (1999) Magic medicine cabinet: a situated portal for consumer healthcare. In proc. of the International Symposium on Handheld and Ubiquitous Computing (HUC '99)

[15] Palen L, Aaløkke S (2006) Of pill boxes and piano benches: "home-made" methods for managing medication. In Proc. of ACM Conference on Computer Supported Collaborative Work (CSCW2006), 79-88, Nov.

[16] Siegemund F, Florkemeier C (2003) Interaction in pervasive computing settings using Bluetooth-enabled active tags and passive RFID technology together with mobile phones. In Proc. of IEEE Conference on Pervasive Computing (Percom03)